Vivian A. Fonseca
Merri Pendergrass
Roberta Harrison McDuffie

Diabetes in Clinical Practice

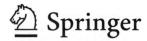 Springer

Vivian A. Fonseca
Tulane University Medical Center
New Orleans
Louisiana
USA

Merri Pendergrass
Harvard Medical School
And
Division of Endocrinology, Diabetes
  and Hypertension
Brigham and Women's Hospital
Boston
Massachusetts
USA

Roberta Harrison McDuffie
Tulane University Health Science
  Center Diabetes Program
New Orleans
Louisiana
USA

ISBN 978-1-84882-102-6   e-ISBN 978-1-84882-103-3
Springer London Dordrecht Heidelberg New York
DOI 10.1007/978-1-84882-103-3

A catalogue record for this book is available from the British Library

Library of Congress Control Number: 2009935337

Previously published in 2006 by Current Medicine Group Ltd. as *Handbook of Diabetes*
(ISBN 978-1-85873-414-9)

Springer is part of Springer Science+Business Media (www.springer.com)

Contents

Author biographies

Vivian A. Fonseca, MD, FRCP, FACE, is Professor of Medicine, the Tullis Tulane Alumni Chair in Diabetes, and Chief of the Section of Endocrinology at Tulane University Medical Center in New Orleans, Louisiana, USA. Dr Fonseca's current research interests include the prevention and treatment of diabetic complications and risk factor reduction in cardiovascular disease. He has a research program evaluating homocysteine and inflammation as risk factors for heart disease in diabetes. He is also an investigator in the National Institutes of Health (NIH)-funded Action to Control Cardiovascular Risk in Diabetes (ACCORD) study.

Dr Fonseca previously served as Chair for the American Diabetes Association (ADA) Clinical Practice Committee and the joint ADA/American College of Cardiology (ACC) "Make the Link" program. He is Editor-in-Chief of *Diabetes Care*, and was Associate Editor of the *Journal of the Metabolic Syndrome and Related Disorders* and is also on the editorial board of the *Journal of Clinical Endocrinology and Metabolism*. He is an ad hoc reviewer for several other journals, including *Diabetes, Diabetic Medicine, Kidney International, American Journal of Clinical Nutrition, Journal of Clinical Endocrinology and Metabolism, British Medical Journal, JAMA*, and *Metabolism*.

Dr Fonseca is a fellow of the American Association of Clinical Endocrinologists, the Royal College of Physicians (London), and the American College of Physicians. He is a member of the Endocrine Society, the American Diabetes Association, and the International Diabetes Federation. He has lectured in the USA and abroad, serves on several national and international committees, and has published more than 100 papers, review articles, and book chapters.

Merri Pendergrass, MD, PhD, is an Associate Professor of Medicine at Harvard Medical School and Director of Clinical Diabetes and Associate Clinical Chief in the Division of Endocrinology, Metabolism and Hypertension at Brigham and Women's Hospital, Boston, MA, USA.

Dr Pendergrass' research focuses on developing and implementing strategies to improve diabetes care in healthcare systems. Current projects include developing effective inpatient glucose management protocols; and using medical informatics techniques to characterize barriers to good diabetes care and to identify potential targets for quality improvement interventions.

Dr Pendergrass is a reviewer for a number of journals including *Diabetes Care, Metabolic Syndrome and Related Disorders*, and *New England Journal of Medicine*; and is on the editorial board for *Nature Clinical Practice Endocrinology & Metabolism* and *Diabetes Care*. She has lectured widely in the USA and abroad, and has published more than 50 clinical papers, review articles, and book chapters.

Roberta Harrison McDuffie, MSN, BSBA, APRN, BC, CNS, CDE, is Clinical Trial Coordinator, Tulane University School of Medicine, Clinical Nurse Specialist in Diabetes, and a Certified Diabetes Educator with her own consulting company, Diabetes Wellness Consulting, Inc. Ms McDuffie is also on the faculty of Tulane University Health Sciences Center.

Type 2 diabetes: the modern epidemic

Type 2 diabetes is a major clinical and public health problem. It is estimated that in the year 2000, 171 million people worldwide had type 2 diabetes, including about 18 million Americans, and it is estimated that these numbers will grow to 366 million people worldwide and 30 million Americans by the year 2030.

This high prevalence of diabetes leads to a high global burden of the condition and its complications. Diabetes is the leading cause of blindness below the age of 65 years, and it is responsible for almost half the cases needing dialysis. It is responsible for most non-traumatic amputations. The financial cost of this condition is staggering, with one in seven healthcare dollars in the USA spent on treating the condition or its complications. Indeed, despite the fact that only about 10–15% of the Medicare population has diabetes, about 25% of the American Medicare budget is spent on this condition. In addition, there is a considerable expenditure on the social costs involved with people who suffer with long-term complications, including disability and premature death.

The purpose of this handbook is to give the practitioner a quick overview of the subject, along with practical suggestions for the management of this condition.

Diagnosing diabetes

Criteria for the diagnosis of diabetes
- Symptoms of diabetes (polyuria, polydipsia, unexplained weight loss) plus random plasma glucose concentration >200 mg/dL (11 mmol/L).
- Fasting plasma glucose (FPG) >126 mg/dL (7 mmol/L) (Fasting = no caloric intake for at least 8 h.)
- Two-hour plasma glucose >200 mg/dL (11 mmol/L) during an oral glucose tolerance test (OGTT) (75 g).

In the absence of unequivocal hyperglycemia with acute metabolic decompensation, these criteria should be confirmed by repeat testing on a different day. The OGTT is not recommended for routine clinical use.

V.A. Fonseca et al., *Diabetes in Clinical Practice*,
DOI 10.1007/978-1-84882-103-3_1, © Springer-Verlag London Limited 2010

These diagnostic criteria are summarized in Figure 1.1.

The diagnosis of diabetes is currently made on the basis of several diagnostic criteria (summarized above) [1]. In patients who have classic symptoms, such as polyuria, polydipsia, and weight loss, a random plasma glucose greater than 200 mg/dL (11 mmol/L) is diagnostic. However, most patients are asymptomatic and those suspected of having diabetes should be screened with either a fasting glucose or a 75 g glucose tolerance test. An FPG greater than or equal to 126 mg/dL (7 mmol/L) is considered diagnostic of diabetes, but should be confirmed on another occasion in asymptomatic patients. Following an OGTT, a value greater than 200 mg/dL (11 mmol/L) is considered diagnostic. However, values below these figures are not entirely normal, as a normal fasting glucose is less than 100 mg/dL (5.5 mmol/L), and therefore fasting glucose between 100 mg/dL (5.5 mmol/L) and 125 mg/dL (7 mmol/L) is diagnostic of impaired fasting glucose (IFG), and a 2-hour post-glucose load of 140–199 mg/dL (7.8–11.0 mmol/L) is called impaired glucose tolerance (IGT). Both of these conditions predict increased risk of subsequent progression to diabetes, and also of macrovascular complications, even in the absence of progression to diabetes. The latter is particularly true in patients with IGT.

It is also relatively easy to identify people who are at increased risk of diabetes, who should therefore be screened early even if asymptomatic in order to start treatment early, or take preventive steps described below should they have IFG or IGT.

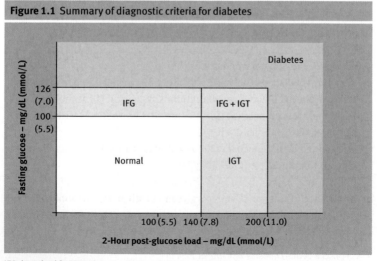

Figure 1.1 Summary of diagnostic criteria for diabetes

IFG, impaired fasting glucose; IGT, impaired glucose tolerance

Who should be screened for diabetes
- Consider testing for all individuals >45 years; if normal, repeat every 3 years
- Consider testing at a younger age or more frequently for high-risk individuals:
- obese (>120% desirable body weight or a body mass index (BMI) >27 kg/m^2)
- having a first-degree relative with diabetes
- members of a high-risk ethnic population (e.g. African-American, Hispanic, Native American)
- delivered a baby weighing >9 lbs (4 kg) or have been diagnosed with gestational diabetes mellitus
- hypertensive (>140/90 mmHg)
- having a high-density lipoprotein cholesterol (HDL-C) level <35 mg/dL and/or a triglyceride level >250 mg/dL (280 mmol/L)
- IGT or IFG on previous testing
- In clinical settings, the FPG is preferred over the OGTT due to ease of administration, convenience, patient acceptability, and lower cost

The diagnostic criteria have been selected on the basis of epidemiologic evidence suggesting that there is a threshold for risk in the development of retinopathy at these levels. However, glucose is a continuous variable in the population, and the relationship with cardiovascular disease (CVD) is almost linear – any increment in glucose leads to an increase in the risk of CVD. This risk is also present even if only the postprandial glucose is elevated and the fasting glucose normal (isolated IGT). Some difficulty arises in differentiating between type 1 diabetes and type 2 diabetes. The distinction is important (*see* Figure 1.2) since insulin is usually critical for life in patients with type 1 diabetes.

While type 1 diabetes often develops in childhood and type 2 diabetes in adults, the reverse can also be true. Similarly, while patients with type 2 diabetes are usually obese, about 10–15% of people may not have obesity, and with the increase in obesity, several patients with type 1 diabetes may actually have type 2 diabetes. Other differentiating features that may help with classification include family history, which is much more common in type 2 diabetes, and also a history of ketoacidosis, which is invariable in type 1 diabetes, although it may occasionally occur in type 2 diabetes. More important, diagnostic markers include the presence of other autoimmune diseases being associated with type 1 diabetes, and the presence of

Figure 1.2 Distinction between types of diabetes

Type 1 diabetes

β-cell destruction, usually leading to absolute insulin deficiency

- Immune mediated
- Idiopathic

Type 2 diabetes

May range from predominantly insulin resistance with relative insulin deficiency to a predominantly secretory defect with insulin resistance

Other specific types

- Genetic defects of β-cell function
- Genetic defects in insulin action
- Diseases of the exocrine pancreas
- Endocrinopathies
- Drug- or chemical-induced
- Infections
- Uncommon forms of immune-mediated diabetes
- Other genetic syndromes sometimes associated with diabetes

Gestational diabetes mellitus

some antibodies, particularly antibodies to glutamic acid decarboxylase (anti-GAD) in type 1. *Figure 1.3* summarizes the differences between type 1 diabetes and type 2 diabetes.

Prediction and prevention of type 2 diabetes

Prediction

Type 2 diabetes can frequently be predicted in patients who have a wide variety of risk factors as summarized above. Patients with these risk factors should be considered for screening at an earlier age than those without these conditions. These include patients with prior IGT or IFG, prior gestational diabetes or polycystic ovarian syndrome, obesity, certain ethnic groups, and patients with known vascular disease and hypertension.

In contrast, prediction of type 1 diabetes is more difficult and currently is not routinely carried out in clinical practice. However, research studies have identified siblings of patients who are at risk based on their HLA type and the presence of islet cell and other antibodies.

Figure 1.3 Summary of the differences between type 1 and type 2 diabetes

	Type 1	Type 2
Age at onset	Usually younger at onset	Usually older, but now seen in adolescents
Weight	~20% overweight	Most overweight
Family history	10% with a close relative	>50% with a close relative
Diabetic ketoacidosis	Frequently in history	Rare
Blood sugars	More variable; severe hypoglycemia	More stable; milder hypoglycemia
Thyroid disease	Often	Sometimes
Treatment	Always insulin	Multiple agents including insulin
Antibodies	Often present (anti-GAD)	Not usually present
Plasma C-peptide/ insulin	Usually low	Early high, later declines

GAD, glutamic acid decarboxylase.

Prevention

Several clinical trials have demonstrated that modest changes in lifestyle may lead to reduction in the risk of new onset diabetes. The most effective treatment that is safe and easily achieved at low cost is lifestyle change, including walking for 30 minutes a day and losing about 5% of body weight. The results of the Diabetes Prevention Program (DPP) (*see* Figures 1.4 and 1.5) demonstrate that intensive lifestyle change resulted in a 58% reduction in the conversion of IGT to diabetes. Metformin reduced the risk by about 30%, being more effective in younger obese subjects. In the DREAM study, ramipril was not effective in preventing diabetes, whereas rosiglitazone led

Figure 1.4 Summary of major diabetes prevention studies

Study	Intervention	Relative risk reduction (%)
Finnish DPS	Diet and exercise	58
Diabetes Prevention Program	Diet and exercise	58
	Metformin	31 (53% if obese)
STOP-NIDDM	Acarbose	36
TRIPOD	Troglitazone	56
DREAM	Rosiglitazone	60
	Ramipril	NS

DPS, Diabetes Prevention Study; DREAM, Diabetes REduction Assessment with ramipril and rosiglitazone Medication; STOP-NIDDM, Study TO Prevent Non-Insulin-Dependent Diabetes Mellitus; TRIPOD, Troglitazone in the Prevention of Diabetes.

to a 60% reduction in conversion to diabetes. However, rosiglitazone was associated with an increased risk of heart failure and is therefore unlikely to be recommended for diabetes prevention. Based on clinical trials so far, the following recommendations in *Figures 1.5–1.7* can be made.

Figure 1.5 Suggested recommendations for prevention of diabetes

Population	Treatment
Impaired fasting glucose or impaired glucose tolerance	Lifestyle modification (i.e. 5–10% weight loss and moderate intensity physical activity ~30 min/day)
Individuals with impaired fasting glucose and impaired glucose tolerance and any of the following: • <60 years of age • BMI >35 kg/m^2 • Family history of diabetes in first-degree relatives • Elevated triglycerides • Reduced HDL cholesterol • Hypertension • Hemoglobin A1C >6.0%	Lifestyle modification (as above) and/or metformin*

* Metformin 850 mg twice per day if no contraindications. Note, metformin is not approved by the FDA for prevention of diabetes. BMI, body mass index; HDL, high-density lipoprotein. Modified with permission from [2].

Figure 1.6 Strategies for prevention of type 2 diabetes

Individuals at high risk for developing diabetes need to become aware of the benefits of modest weight loss and participating in regular physical activity.

Patients with IGT should be given counseling on weight loss as well as instruction for increasing physical activity.

Patients with IFG should be given counseling on weight loss as well as instruction for increasing physical activity.

Follow-up counseling appears important for success.

Monitoring for the development of diabetes in those with pre-diabetes should be performed every 1–2 years.

Close attention should be given to, and appropriate treatment given for, other CVD risk factors (e.g. tobacco use, hypertension, dyslipidemia).

Drug therapy should not be routinely used to prevent diabetes as the drugs are not approved for this indication. However, metformin could be used cautiously in selected patients.

CVD, cardiovascular disease; IFG, impaired fasting glucose; IGT, impaired glucose tolerance.

Figure 1.7 Suggested algorithm for preventing diabetes

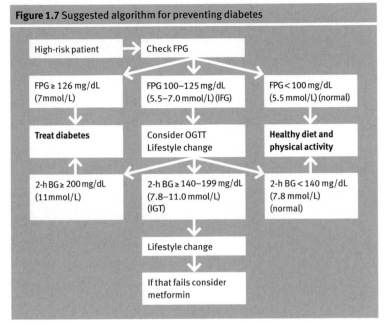

Note: metformin and other medications have not been approved for prevention.
BG, blood glucose; FPG, fasting plasma glucose; IFG, impaired fasting glucose;
IGT, impaired glucose tolerance; OGTT, oral glucose tolerance test.

References

1 American Diabetes Association. Standards of medical care in diabetes – 2007. Diabetes Care 2007; 30 (Suppl 1):S4–S41.
2 Nathan DM, Davidson MB, DeFronzo RA, et al. Impaired fasting glucose and impaired glucose tolerance: implications for care. Diabetes Care 2007: 30(3):753–759.

Chapter 2

Management of diabetes

Goals of treatment

Historically, patient treatment has been *reactive*, guided by the assessment of patients' symptoms. However, elevated blood glucose, elevated blood pressure and elevated cholesterol often have no symptoms. Yet, research has demonstrated that early and successful treatment of these problems can prevent or delay complications of diabetes [1].

In the long-term, treatment goals of diabetes are intended to prevent microvascular complications, including blindness, kidney failure and amputations, and, to whatever extent possible, prevent macrovascular complications as well. The healthcare provider's goal for the diabetes patient must be *proactive*, working to extend life while maximizing wellness for the individual patient, based on the patient's informed choice of treatment goals. In the short term, the healthcare provider can be guided by treatment goals established by a variety of experts. Experts recommend that the primary focus of the providers' attention be on controlling the ABCs of diabetes: A1C, blood pressure and cholesterol [2] (*see* Figure 2.1).

To further facilitate achievement of treatment goals, a treatment plan for diabetes patients should include those assessments necessary to evaluate patient progress toward achieving long-term goals (*see* Figure 2.2). The hemoglobin A1C test, available also as a point of care test, can be used to help engage patients in discussions of treatment goals as well as to facilitate collaborative agreements on treatment plan changes that are needed to achieve the desired treatment goals [4].

The healthcare provider should be aware of the importance of negotiating and achieving agreement with the patient regarding the diabetes treatment plan. Stronger provider–patient agreements on treatment plans and strategies for achieving treatment goals correlates well with improved patient self-efficacy and diabetes self-management [5].

V.A. Fonseca et al., *Diabetes in Clinical Practice*,
DOI 10.1007/978-1-84882-103-3_2, © Springer-Verlag London Limited 2010

Figure 2.1 A summary of recommendations for adults
with diabetes

Goals for glycemic control

Hemoglobin A1C	< 7%
Preprandial glucose	90–130 mg/dL (5.0–7.2 mmol/L)
2 h postprandial glucose	< 180 mg/dL (<10 mmol/L)

Goals for lipids

Low-density lipoprotein	< 100 mg/dL (<2.6 mmol/L)
Triglycerides	< 150 mg/dL (<1.7 mmol/L)
High-density lipoprotein	> 40 mg/dL (>1.0 mmol/L)

Goals for blood pressure	< 130/80 mmHg

Adapted from [3].

Figure 2.2 Assessment guidelines

Every visit
Blood pressure
Weight
Visual foot examination

Quarterly
Hemoglobin A1C

Biannual
Dental examination

Annually
Albumin/creatinine ratio (unless proteinuria is documented)
Pedal pulses and neurologic examination
Dilated eye examination (by trained expert)
Examine patient for factors linked to clinical depression
Blood lipids
Assessment of diabetes knowledge and ability to provide self-care, including:
  self monitoring blood glucose (SMBG)
  meal planning and nutrition
  physical activity
  weight management

Data from [3].

A chronic care model that is well-fitted to individual practices m; able in assisting patients to achieve appropriate treatment goals. Readi well-organized patient information and use of health information provide additional assistance [6]. One frequently used model, the Chronic Care Model, developed by the MacColl Institute, is shown in *Figure 2.3*.

Shared care – the multidisciplinary approach

In the midst of the current diabetes epidemic, there appears to be consensus by diabetes experts on the need for a team approach to diabetes management and education [8]. A report by the American Association of Clinical Endocrinologists (AACE) indicated that two out of three patients with type 2 diabetes do not have hemoglobin A1C levels under control. Nevertheless, in a related survey reported by AACE, 84% of patients reported that their blood glucose levels were "well controlled" [9] which begs the conclusion that many patients do not understand the values associated with "good control". Patients need high quality, up-to-date diabetes education, as part of a formal education process, as well as continuing education, as part of every visit with each of the team members. These educational opportunities will provide patients with all of the information necessary for skilled diabetes self-management, including development of treatment goals.

The National Diabetes Education Program provides a detailed plan to assist providers in developing a functional multidisciplinary team capable of providing patients with consistent, aggressive treatment as well as educational opportunities that will meet the individual needs of patients while assisting

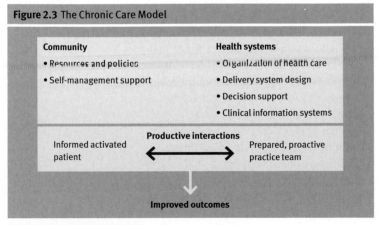

Figure 2.3 The Chronic Care Model

Community
• Resources and policies
• Self-management support

Health systems
• Organization of health care
• Delivery system design
• Decision support
• Clinical information systems

Informed activated patient

Productive interactions

←——————————→

Prepared, proactive practice team

Improved outcomes

Adapted with permission from [7].

patients to achieve the most appropriate therapeutic goal desired by the patient [10] (*see* Figure 2.4).

Healthy eating and weight control

Recommendations for healthy eating and weight control
- Eat a well-balanced, wide variety of foods
- Eat 2–4 daily servings of fruits
- Eat 3–5 daily servings of vegetables
- Limit salt, alcohol, saturated fats, cholesterol, foods containing sugar and fast foods
- Eat smaller portions and never skip meals
- Choose whole grain foods whenever possible
- Consult with a diabetes educator and/or registered dietitian for assistance in preparing an individualized meal plan. Carbohydrate counting, as a meal-planning alternative, can be discussed at this meeting, if desired.

General goals of medical nutrition therapy (MNT) for diabetes
- MNT should facilitate achievement of metabolic goals including glucose levels, lipid levels and blood pressure levels that minimizes a patient's risks of microvascular and macrovascular complications related to diabetes.
- MNT should be appropriate for optimum management of existing diabetes complications and risk factors for further complications.
- MNT should facilitate attainment of the maximum level of wellness for each individual
- MNT should be tailored to meet the personal needs of each patient [13].

Studies suggest that approximately 80% of people with type 2 diabetes are overweight or obese [14]. Experts agree that people with type 2 diabetes should be encouraged to achieve and maintain a desirable body weight. A majority of these experts agree with the following recommendations:
- a body mass index (BMI) of <25 kg/m²;
- carbohydrates as 50–60% of intake;
- protein intake of 11–18% of total calories;
- limiting fat to 25–30% of calorie intake;
- fiber intake of 25–35 g/day;
- use of low glycemic index foods;
- use of whole grains, legumes, vegetables and fruits [15].

Significant research has been done to confirm the correlation between weight loss and improved insulin sensitivity as well as improved glycemic control

Figure 2.4 Diabetes healthcare team members

Patient
"Expert"; personal abilities,
"feelings", "monitor" of: food,
exercise, glucose

Nurse educator
Has specialized training in
diabetes, teaches day-to-
day management skills

Primary care provider
Focused on patient-
centered care and
well-trained in diabetes
treatment and medication
regimens

Registered dietitian
Trained and certified with
experience in diabetes

Social worker
Deals with
the emotions
related to living
with chronic
disease

Eye doctor
Evaluates
eye health
annually

Dentist
Evaluates
dental health
biannually

Podiatrist
Treats corns,
calluses as well
as other foot
problems

**Excercise
physiologist**
Assists in
planning fitness
programs that
will help provide
efficiency
in diabetes
management

Cardiologist, nephrologist, neurologist, pharmacist, pedorthist / orthotist

Community support: church groups, support groups, employer support

Note
Strategies for successful diabetes team management:
- The patient should be the team leader. This is a critical concept due to the chronic
  nature of the disease. It requires lifelong self-management. Achievement of treatment
  goals depends significantly on patient commitment to those goals.
- Patient self-management education should be an ongoing process consisting of both
  formal and informal processes. The quality of patient education will be a determining
  factor in patient outcomes.
- The Diabetes Team should consistently act to facilitate achievement of treatment
  goals.
- All team members should maintain current and consistent knowledge of the disease,
  the treatment process, the goals of treatment and the education and management
  processes that facilitate those goals.
- Alternating visits between physicians and nurse practitioners.
- Routine nurse phone assessments of glycemic control.
- Dietitian visits for patients.

Data from [3, 8, 11, 12].

[16]. There are a number of strategies that can be encouraged to improve overall nutrition, facilitating weight loss. Among those are [17]:
• food logs that include all food intake over specified periods of time;
• nutritional counseling to improve meal planning and food choices as well as information on portion sizes;
• behavioral counseling to improve stimulus control;
• structured weight loss diets; and
• meal replacements.

In a recent study, significant improvement in A1C of 1.0–1.6 ± 0.3–0.4% related to an approximate 10% weight loss were achieved without use of antihyperglycemic pharmacologic interventions [18]. One study found that a maximum reduction in hyperglycemia of approximately 87% occurred during the first 10 days of a calorie-restricted diet, even though only a small percentage of weight loss had occurred [19]. The findings of a recent study by Kelley, *et al.* indicate that a short period of calorie restriction can result

Figure 2.5 The Food Pyramid

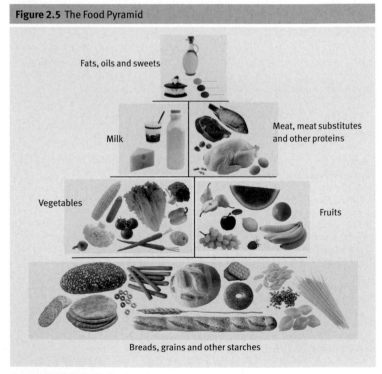

Reproduced with permission from [21].

in significant improvements in insulin sensitivity, insulin secretion and hepatic glucose production, supporting the theory that total daily calories may exert the greatest impact on glucose homeostasis in patients with type 2 diabetes [20].

Nutrition recommendations should be based on the Food Pyramid (*see* Figure 2.5) which allows for variations in the appropriate number of servings as determined by individual evaluations including nutritional status, likes and dislikes, and other health issues.

Exercise

A recently released study revealed that the majority of patients with type 2 diabetes do not perform regular exercise or physical activities – in fact, they engage in physical activity at a rate much below national norms [22]. A recent meta-analysis of 27 studies to evaluate various types of exercise including aerobic, resistance, and combined training exercise, in a total of 1003 patients with type 2 diabetes, determined that all forms of exercise training produce small benefits in A1C, the main measure of glucose control. Benefits were similar to those achieved with dietary and pharmaceutical treatments [23]. Exercise actually includes all physical activities, even routine work such as mowing the lawn (pushing a mower), gardening or cleaning the house (*see* Figure 2.6). The benefits of physical activity include:

- reduction of blood glucose levels;
- reduction of blood pressure levels;
- reduction of cholesterol levels;
- reduction of cardiovascular risks for heart attack and stroke;
- reduction of stress;
- improved muscle tone, including heart muscle;
- improved bone strength;
- improved flexibility;
- improved blood circulation; and
- weight loss.

A study of Finnish adults with type 2 diabetes demonstrated that both a moderate as well as a high level of exercise are associated with a decreased risk of total and cardiovascular mortality. The positive association between exercise and longevity occurred regardless of BMI, blood pressure readings, total cholesterol levels and smoking [25]. Exercise recommendations should include a 5–10 minute warm up and a similar cool down period as well as a pre-exercise stretching period of 5–10 minutes. Blood glucose should be checked before exercise.

Figure 2.6 Calories burned during exercise

Activities (1 hour)	Calories burned according to weight	
	140–150 lbs (64–68 kg)	170–180 lbs (77–82 kg)
Aerobic dancing	416–442	501–533
Bicycling	512–544	616–656
Bowling	192–204	231–246
Dancing	288–306	347–369
Gardening	256–272	308–328
Golfing (carrying bag)	288–306	347–369
Jogging (5 mph)	512–544	616–656
Stair climbing	576–612	693–738
Swimming	384–408	462–492
Tennis	448–476	539–574
Walking (2 mph)	160–170	193–205
Walking (3.5 mph)	243–258	293–312

Adapted from [24].

In discussions with patients regarding exercise, the following issues should be considered [26]:
- maintaining proper hydration;
- wearing proper footwear;
- monitoring feet well for blisters and other types of damage;
- diabetes identification should be worn at all times; and
- treatment for hypoglycemia should be carried at all times, preferably glucose tablets.

For each individual, their exercise program should be well thought-out and take into account:
- type of exercise;
- intensity;
- duration;
- frequency;
- rate of progression;
- when to check blood glucose;
- how to adjust medications; and
- plan for follow-up.

The healthcare provider should evaluate the patient for any signs and symptoms of heart and/or blood vessel disease, eye disease, nervous system disorders, kidney disease and specific foot problems. Special exercise considerations are required for patients with these particular disorders [27].

References

1 Phillips LS, Branch WT, Cook CB, et al. Clinical inertia. Ann Intern Med 2001; 135(9):825–834.

2 The National Diabetes Education Program. Working together to manage diabetes: a guide for pharmacy, podiatry, optometry, and dental professionals. Available at: http://ndep. nih.gov/diabetes/pubs/PPODprimer_color.pdf. Last accessed September 2007.

3 American Diabetes Association. Standards of medical care in diabetes. Diabetes Care 2007; 30(Suppl 1):S4–S41.

4 Delamater AM. Clinical use of hemoglobin A1c to improve diabetes management. Clin Diabetes 2006; 24:6–8.

5 Heisler M, Vijan S, Anderson RM, et al. When do patients and their physicians agree on diabetes treatment goals and strategies, and what difference does it make? J Gen Intern Med 2003; 18(11):893–902.

6 Bergenstal, RM. Overcoming clinical inertia in diabetes care. Physician's Weekly 2007; 24:1–2.

7 Wagner EH. Chronic disease management: what will it take to improve care for chronic illness? Eff Clin Pract 1998; 1(1):2–4.

8 Landers, SJ. Team effort best way to control diabetes. Available at: www.ama-assn.org/ amednews/site/free/hlsb0703.htm. Last accessed September 2007.

9 American Association of Clinical Endocrinologists. State of diabetes in America: a new report reveals America's diabetes health is in jeopardy. Available at: www.aace.com/ newsroom/press/2005/index.php/r=20050518_2. Last accessed September 2007.

10 The National Diabetes Education Program. Team care: comprehensive lifetime management for diabetes. Available at: http://ndep.nih.gov/diabetes/pubs/TeamCare.pdf. Last accessed September 2007.

11 Miller CD, Phillips LS, Tate MK, et al. Meeting American Diabetes Association guidelines in endocrinologist practice. Diabetes Care 2000; 23(4):444–448.

12 Piette JD, Weinberger M, McPhee SJ, et al. Do automated calls with nurse follow-up improve elf-care and glycemic control among vulnerable patients with diabetes? Am J Med 2000; 108(1):20–27.

13 American Diabetes Association. Position Statement: Nutrition Principles and Recommendations in Diabetes. Diabetes Care 2004; 27(Suppl 1):S36.

14 Hensrud DD. Dietary Treatment and Long-Term Weight Loss and maintenance in Type 2 Diabetes. Obes Res 2001; 9(Suppl 4):348S–353S

15 Anderson JW, Randles KM, Kendall CWC, Jenkins DJA. Carbohydrate and fiber recommendations for individuals with diabetes: a quantitative assessment and meta-analysis of the evidence. J Am Coll Nutr 2004; 23(1):5–17

16 Ferrannini E, Camastra S, Gastaldelli A, Sironi AM, et al. Beta cell function in obesity: effects of weight loss. Diabetes 2004; 53:S26–33.

17 Franz MJ, Bantle JP, Beebe CA, et al. Evidence-based nutrition principles and recommendations for the treatment and prevention of diabetes and related complications. Diabetes Care 2002; 25(1):148–98.

18 Kelley DE, Kuller LH, McKolanis TM, et al. Effects of moderate weight loss and orlistat on insulin resistance, regional adiposity, and fatty acids in type 2 diabetes. Diabetes Care 2004; 27(1):33–40

19 Henry RR, Scheaffer L, Olefsky JM. Glycemic effects of intensive caloric restriction and isocaloric refeeding in noninsulin-dependent diabetes mellitus. J Clin Endocrinol Metab 1985; 61:917–925.

20 Kelley DE, Wing R, Buonocore C, et al. Relative effects of calorie restriction and weight loss in noninsulin-dependent diabetes mellitus. J Clin Endocrinol Metab 1993; 77(5):1287–1293.

21 American Diabetes Association. Using the Diabetes Food Pyramid. Available at: http://diabetes. org/nutrition-and-recipes/nutrition/foodpyramid.jsp. Last accessed September 2007.

22 Morrato EH, Hill JO, Wyatt HR, Ghushchyan V, Sullivan PW. Physical activity in U.S. adults with diabetes and at risk for developing diabetes, 2003. Diabetes Care 2007; 30(2):203–9.

23 Snowling NJ, Hopkins WG. Effects of different modes of exercise training on glucose control and risk factors for complications in type 2 diabetic patients: a meta-analysis. Diabetes Care 2006; 29(11):2518–27.

24 Exercise: Calories burned in 1 hour of exercise. Available at: www.mayoclinic.com/health/exercise/SM00109. Last accessed September 2007.

25 Hu G, Jousilahti P, Barengo NC, Qiao Q, Lakka TA, Tuomilehto J. Physical activity, cardiovascular risk factors, and mortality among Finnish adults with diabetes. Diabetes Care 2005; 28(4):799–805.

26 American Diabetes Association. Diabetes mellitus and exercise: position statement. Diabetes Care 2002; 25:S64.

27 American Diabetes Association. Physical activity/exercise and diabetes mellitus. Diabetes Care 2003; 26:S73–S77.

Chapter 3

Non-insulin agents in the management of type 2 diabetes

Eight different classes of medication, in addition to insulin, are currently approved for treatment of hyperglycemia in type 2 diabetes. Beneficial effects of antihyperglycemic agents appear to be mediated predominantly through their ability to lower blood glucose. Studies are currently in progress to determine whether any particular agent (or treatment strategy) has specific advantages, beyond glucose lowering, in terms of reducing cardiovascular endpoints [1, 2].

Unfortunately, there are few high quality head-to-head comparison trials evaluating the ability of available non-insulin agents to achieve recommended glycemic targets. This is important, since the glucose-lowering effectiveness of individual medications is strongly influenced by baseline characteristics such as A1C level, duration of diabetes and previous therapy. With these limitations in mind, the relative glucose-lowering effectiveness of available agents is outlined in *Figure 3.1*.

Until recently, there have been no widely accepted treatment guidelines for which medicines to prescribe and in what sequence. A recent American Diabetes Association (ADA) and European Association for the Study of

Figure 3.1 Effectiveness of agents on A1C levels

Class (example)	Approximate A1C reduction (%)
Biguanidoe (metformin)	0.9–2.5
Sulfonylureas (glipizide, glyburide, glimiperide, others)	1.1–3.0
Glinides (repaglinide, nateglindide)	1.0–1.5
Thiazolidinediones (pioglitazone, rosiglitazone)	1.5–1.6
α-Glucosidase inhibitors (acarbose, miglitol)	0.6–1.3
Gliptins (sitagliptin)	0.8
GLP-1 analogs (exenetide)	0.8–0.9
Amylin analogs (pramlintide)	0.4–0.6

GLP-1, glucagon-like peptide 1. Data from [13, 14, 33].

V.A. Fonseca et al., *Diabetes in Clinical Practice*,
DOI 10.1007/978-1-84882-103-3_3, © Springer-Verlag London Limited 2010

Diabetes (EASD) consensus statement recommended a treatment algorithm promoting preferential use of older, less expensive agents including metformin, sulfonylureas, and insulin [3]. This recommendation was consistent with findings of another recent report that concluded that, compared with newer agents, sulfonylureas and metformin have similar or superior effects on glycemic control, lipids, and other intermediate end points [4]. It is too early to determine what the effect of these guidelines will have on prescribing practices. Diabetes treatment is extremely complex; decisions are typically individualized based on multiple factors that may be weighted differently in the guidelines than in clinical practice. Physicians make treatment decisions based on their clinical assessments of their patients' health and comorbid conditions, adherence, tendency to experience side effects, motivation to improve and/or avoid insulin and many other factors [5]. Decisions also may be influenced by formulary restrictions, as well as costs.

In summary, no single treatment strategy has been shown to be superior for all patients. Decisions about which medication or combination of medications to use should be made based on their effects on A1C levels, contraindications, side-effect profiles, patient preferences, and expense.

In this chapter we begin by briefly reviewing glycemic treatment goals and pathogenesis of hyperglycemia in type 2 diabetes. We then summarize features of each of the non-insulin therapies and highlight potential advantages and disadvantages of available treatment options. We conclude with discussions on how to select an initial therapy and how to optimize combinations of agents.

Treatment goals

The A1C is the primary target for glycemic control. The goal of therapy is to achieve an A1C as close to normal as possible without unacceptable levels of hypoglycemia. Postprandial glucose may be targeted if A1C goals are not met despite reaching preprandial glucose goals. Although an A1C of below 7% is recommended for most patients, available data do not identify the optimal level of control for individual patients. Less stringent goals may be appropriate for patients with limited life expectancies or significant comorbidities. More stringent goals may be indicated for younger, healthier, and/or pregnant patients.

Pathogenesis of hyperglycemia in type 2 diabetes

Type 2 diabetes is a heterogeneous disease manifested by hyperglycemia that results from multiple dysregulated biologic pathways. Each of these pathways represents a potential target for therapy (*see Figure 3.2*). The two major metabolic abnormalities are: 1) insulin resistance in skeletal muscle, liver, and adipocytes, and 2) a progressive decline in insulin production by

Figure 3.2 Effect of agents on the biologic pathways in patients with type 2 diabetes

Class	Primary mechanism of action
Biguanides	Decrease glucose production (liver)
Sulfonylureas	Increase insulin secretion (pancreas)
Glinides	Increase insulin secretion (pancreas)
Thiazolidinediones	Increase glucose uptake (muscle, fat)
α-Glucosidase inhibitors	Delay carbohydrate absorption (gut)
Gliptins	Prolong effects of GLP-1 (↑ insulin,↓ glucagon)
GLP-1 analogs	Similar effects as GLP-1 (↑ insulin,↓ glucagon,↑ satiety, delays gastric emptying)
Amylin analogs	Similar effects as amylin (↓ glucagon,↑ satiety, delays gastric emptying)

GLP-1, glucagon-like peptide 1; ↑, increased; ↓, decreased.

pancreatic β-cells [6]. Insulin resistance results from both environmental factors (predominantly obesity and physical inactivity) and genetic factors that have yet to be fully identified. Early in the natural history of type 2 diabetes, insulin-resistant individuals who are prediabetic compensate by secreting increased amounts of insulin. Hyperglycemia results as the capacity of the pancreas to secrete insulin deteriorates and endogenous insulin production is insufficient to overcome insulin resistance. Because β-cell failure is progressive, treatment interventions must be continuously monitored and advanced. The progressive β-cell deterioration of type 2 diabetes mandates the stepwise addition of non-insulin agents and/or insulin over time. An agent that could halt the decline in β-cell function, therefore, would be of tremendous benefit. To date, no agent has been definitively shown to do this.

There is increasing evidence that the incretin system may also play a role in glucose homeostasis [7]. The incretin hormone most strongly implicated is glucagon-like peptide 1 (GLP-1). GLP-1 is a naturally occurring peptide produced by the L-cells of the small intestine. Although GLP-1 secretion is reduced in patients with type 2 diabetes, its action is preserved. GLP-1 enhances glucose-dependent insulin secretion, suppresses glucagon secretion, slows gastric emptying, and increases satiety. In normal conditions, GLP-1 is very rapidly cleaved and inactivated by the enzyme dipeptidyl peptidase IV (DPP-IV), which makes native GLP-1 impractical for use as a diabetes treatment. However, other strategies to prolong GLP-1 action, including GLP-1 analogs resistant to DPP-IV inactivation and inhibitors of DPP-IV (*see* below), have been developed as antihyperglycemic agents.

Finally, there is some evidence that amylin, a pancreatic hormone that is normally co-secreted with insulin, may contribute to glucose homeostasis, particularly in advanced type 2 diabetes [8]. Its secretion appears to be diminished in advanced type 2 diabetes, but its action is preserved. Amylin has been found to slow gastric emptying, suppress postprandial glucagon secretion, and increase satiety.

Non-insulin antihyperglycemic agents

Figures 3.3 and 3.4 outline the mechanism of action, dosing characteristics, contraindications, side effects, and costs of available non-insulin therapies. Each class of medications is briefly described below.

Figure 3.3 Prescribing considerations

Class	Dosing characteristics Route	Frequency	Primary contraindications	Common side effects	Effect on body weight
Biguanides	Oral	Once or twice daily	Creatinine > 1.5 man, > 1.4 woman Acute illness	Diarrhea	Decreases
Sulfonylureas	Oral	Once or twice daily	Predisposition to hypoglycemia	Hypoglycemia	Increases
Glinides	Oral	Three times daily before meals			
Thiazolidinediones	Oral	Once or twice daily	ALT >2.5 times ULN CHF (NYHA class III or IV)	Edema, CHF	Increases
α-Glucosidase inhibitors	Oral	Three times daily before meals	Chronic intestinal disorders Cirrhosis Serum creatinine >2.0	Flatulence	Neutral
Gliptins	Oral	Once daily	None	Rare	Neutral
GLP-1 analogs	Parenteral	Twice daily before meals	Severe renal insufficiency (CrCl <30 ml/min)	Nausea	Decreases
Amylin analogs	Parenteral	Three times daily, before meals	Gastroparesis	Nausea	Decreases

ALT, alanine transaminase; CHF, congestive heart failure; CrCl, creatinine clearance; GLP-1, glucagon-like peptide 1; NYHA, New York Heart Association; ULN, upper limit of normal.

Figure 3.4 Cost of therapy

Class	Cost*
Sulfonylureas	$
Biguanides	$
α-Glucosidase inhibitors	$$
Glinides	$$
Thiazolidinediones	$$$
Gliptins	$$$
GLP-1 analogs	$$$
Amylin analogs	$$$

*On a scale where $ indicates least expensive and $$$ indicates most expensive. GLP-1, glucagon-like peptide 1.

Biguanides

Metformin, the only biguanide available, works primarily by decreasing hepatic glucose production. It has been available in other countries since 1957 and in the USA since 1995. It is currently the most widely prescribed diabetes agent in the USA. Metformin has the advantages of not causing hypoglycemia and being associated with weight loss. Although it was found in the United Kingdom Prospective Diabetes Study (UKPDS) to have a beneficial effect on CVD outcomes [9], this finding needs to be confirmed before metformin can be recommended for reduction of cardiovascular risk. The most common adverse effects are gastrointestinal. Lactic acidosis, a potentially fatal adverse effect, is extremely rare, and is associated almost exclusively with other risk factors such as renal or hepatic disease.

Sulfonylureas

Sulfonylureas (SUs) initially became available in the 1940s and have remained a cornerstone of therapy ever since. SUs reduce blood glucose levels by stimulating insulin secretion by the pancreatic β-cells. The combination of their proven efficacy, low incidence of adverse events, and low cost has contributed to their success and continued use. First generation SUs (acetohexamide, chlorpropamide, tolbutamide) should not be used due to increased risk of hypoglycemia and drug interactions. Second generation SUs (glipizide, glyburide, and glimiperide) are frequently used as first-line agents. Sustained-release products offer no advantage over generic, immediate-release SUs, and may be associated with increased rates of nocturnal hypoglycemia.

Back-to-back comparisons between metformin and SUs reveal similar A1C reductions [10]. The major adverse side effect of sulfonylureas is hypoglycemia, which appears to occur most frequently in the elderly. Fortunately, severe episodes tend to be rare. A weight gain of ~2 kg is common with sulfonylurea therapy, which potentially could have an adverse impact on CVD risk. However, increased CVD risk with sulfonylureas has not been established. An early study, The University Group Diabetes Project [11], suggested increased cardiovascular mortality in patients randomized to SUs compared to other oral agents or insulin. This finding was not confirmed in the SU-treated cohort of the more recent UKPDS trial [12].

Glinides
Two agents, repaglinide and nateglinide, are available in the glinide class. Like SUs, they stimulate insulin secretion by binding to the SU receptor. They have a more rapid onset and shorter duration of action than the SUs and are designed to target postprandial hyperglycemia. They should be taken just prior to meals. Repaglinide is similarly effective at A1C reduction as metformin and the SUs [13], while nateglinide is less effective [14]. Compared to SUs, the risk for hypoglycemia is similar with repaglinide but less frequent with nateglinide. Glinides are not commonly used in the USA, most likely because of their higher cost, more frequent dosing, and reduced efficacy (nateglinide) compared to SUs.

Thiazolidinediones
Two thiazolidinediones (TZDs or glitazones), rosiglitazone and pioglitazone, are currently available [15]. They improve glycemia primarily by increasing insulin-mediated glucose uptake in muscle and adipocytes. To a lesser extent, they decrease hepatic glucose production. Compared to SUs and metformin, TZDs are somewhat less effective at lowering blood glucose. Like metformin, TZDs do not cause hypoglycemia when used as monotherapy. The major side effects of TZDs are weight gain and fluid retention. The fluid retention typically manifests as peripheral edema, although new or worsened congestive heart failure can occur. There has been considerable interest regarding the effect of TZDs on cardiovascular risk. Some [16], but not all [17], studies have suggested that rosiglitazone may worsen cardiovascular outcomes. Clinical trial data suggests that pioglitazone may have cardiovascular benefits [18]. Studies that are currently in progress will further help to determine the effects of TZDs on CVD risk [1, 2]. Finally, concerns have also been raised that both rosiglitazone [19] and pioglitazone [20] may increase the risk of fracture, a complication that is already increased in patients with diabetes [21].

Although glitazones are currently used extensively in the USA, given increasing concerns regarding cardiac safety and risk of fracture, known risks of weight gain and congestive heart failure, and high costs, these agents probably should be avoided in patients treated with insulin, those with a history of coronary heart disease, those with congestive heart failure, and those with an increased risk of fracture.

α-Glucosidase inhibitors

Acarbose and miglitol are the two agents in the α-glucosidase inhibitor (AGI) class of antihyperglycemic compounds. AGIs reduce the rate of digestion of polysaccharides in the proximal small intestine. When used before meals, they delay the absorption of complex carbohydrates and blunt postprandial hyperglycemia, resulting in modest reductions in A1C. They are not associated with weight changes or hypoglycemia. AGIs are infrequently used in the USA. The main limitations to their widespread use are the need for frequent dosing, poor tolerability due to frequent gastrointestinal side effects, and only modest antihyperglycemic effects.

GLP-1 analogs

Exenetide is the first member of a new class of agents, the GLP-1 analogs, which affects the incretin system. Because it resists degradation by DPP-IV, it has a significantly longer half-life than GLP-1. Exenatide exhibits many of the same glucoregulatory properties of GLP-1. It enhances glucose-dependent insulin secretion, suppresses hepatic glucagon secretion, slows gastric emptying and reduces food intake. Intriguing results in animal studies suggest that exenatide may also preserve β-cell function.

Although only modest improvements in glycemic control have been demonstrated with exenatide [22], two features make this agent a potentially attractive treatment option. It does not cause hypoglycemia and is associated with about 2–3 kg weight loss. The major limitations to its widespread use are the relatively high frequency of gastrointestinal side effects and the requirement for twice-daily injections. Similar new agents in this class, including a preparation that will require only a single daily (liraglutide, a human GLP-1 analog) or a single weekly injection (long-acting release exenatide), are currently being evaluated in clinical trials. Since exenatide only has been available since June 2005, it is too soon to predict its eventual role in clinical practice.

Dipeptidyl peptidase IV inhibitors

The newest class of antihyperglycemic agents to be approved is the DPP-IV inhibitor. Sitagliptin is the only agent in this classss that is currently approved in the USA. Another agent, vildagliptin, is undergoing Food and Drug Administration (FDA) review. By inhibiting the enzyme DPP-IV, the enzyme that normally inactivates GLP-1, these agents prolong the glucoregulatory actions of GLP-1 [23]. DPP-IV inhibitors modestly reduce A1C levels, are generally very well tolerated, are not associated with hypoglycemia, and are weight neutral [22]. Despite these attractive properties, which have been demonstrated in short-term studies, the long-term effects of these agents remain unknown. DPP-IV is present in other multiple biological systems, including ones involved in immunity and other hormones. This raises the theoretical risk that inhibition of DPP-IV may adversely affect functioning of other systems.

Amylin mimetics

Pramlintide is a synthetic analog of amylin, a hormone that is synthesized by pancreatic β-cells and co-secreted with insulin in response to a meal. Treatment, which requires injections before each meal, is associated with mild reductions in A1C and weight loss [24]. Nausea is a common side effect. These agents are rarely used to treat hyperglycemia in type 2 diabetes.

Selection of initial antihyperglycemic agents

Choice of initial therapy is complex and depends on multiple factors including the patient's initial A1C, the agent's effect on glucose-lowering, cost, side effects, contraindications, dosing frequency, and acceptability to patients. Initial treatment for most patients is a single oral agent, although insulin may be preferred if the patient has very high initial blood glucose levels, is underweight, losing weight, or is ketotic (*see* Figure 3.5). Metformin, SUs, and TZDs are the most commonly used first-line agents, although the role for TZDs may change given increasing safety concerns. From a practical standpoint, glinides, AGIs, pramlintide, exenetide and gliptins are seldom used as first-line agents due low glucose-lowering potential, poor patient tolerability, and/or the need for injection.

There is an emerging consensus that, as long as there are no contraindications, metformin should be initiated, concurrent with lifestyle intervention, at the time of diabetes diagnosis. This opinion was recently published as a joint consensus guideline of the ADA and the EASD [3]. The recommendation is based on the fact that patient adherence with diet, weight reduction, and regular exercise is not sustained in most patients, and most patients will ultimately require treatment. Early institution of treatment for diabetes, at a time when the A1C is not significantly elevated, has been associated with improved glycemic control over time and decreased long-term complications [25]. Since metformin is usually well-tolerated, does not cause hypoglycemia, has favorable effects on

Figure 3.5 Potential treatment algorithm for patients with diabetes

Therapy	Advantages	Disadvantages
Initial therapy		
Recommended		
Decrease body weight and increase physical activity	Improves CVD risk factors	Difficult to achieve and maintain
AND		
Metformin (Choose if no contraindications)	No hypoglycemia Weight loss/neutral Inexpensive	GI side effects
Alternative to metformin		
Insulin (Choose if very hyperglycemic, ketotic, thin and/or losing weight)	Most effective Relatively inexpensive	Injections Monitoring Hypoglycemia Weight gain
OR		
See recommended second agents		
Second agent (in addition to intial therapy)		
Recommended		
Sulfonylurea	Inexpensive	Hypoglycemia Weight gain
OR		
GLP-1 analog	No hypoglycemia Weight loss	Injections GI side effects Expensive
OR		
Gliptin	No hypoglycemia	Limited long-term data Expensive
OR		
Thiazolidinedione	No hypoglycemia	Weight gain CHF Increased fracture risk Possible increased CVD risk Expensive
Alternative		
Insulin (Choose if very hyperglycemic, ketotic, thin and/or losing weight)	See above	See above
Third agent (in addition to above)		
Recommended		
Insulin	See above	See above
Alternative		
Choose additional recommended second agent	See above	See above

CHF, congestive heart failure; CVD, cardiovascular disease; GI, gastrointestinal; GLP-1 glucagon-like peptide 1.

body weight, and is relatively inexpensive, potential benefits of early initiation of medication appear to outweigh potential risks.

Combination therapy

Even if oral agent monotherapy is initially effective, glycemic control is likely to deteriorate over time due to progressive loss of β-cell function in type 2 diabetes. Although metformin is generally recommended as first-line therapy, there is no consensus as to what the second-line agent should be. Numerous two-drug combinations have been studied and have been found to be effective [10, 26–28]. Selection of a second agent, from a different class to the first agent, should be made based on potential advantages and disadvantages. If patients progress to the point where dual therapy does not provide adequate control, either a third non-insulin agent or insulin can be added. In patients with modestly elevated A1C level (below ~8%), addition of a third non-insulin agent may be equally effective as addition of insulin [26, 29, 30]. In this situation, addition of a non-insulin agent may have the advantage of being associated with less weight gain than insulin. For example, exenatide may cause weight loss when used in addition to other oral agents [30]. On the other hand, addition of a third non-insulin agent is likely to be more expensive than addition of insulin [31]. Patients with significantly elevated A1C levels on two non-insulin agents usually should have insulin added to their regimens. A potential treatment algorithm is outlined in *Figure 3.5*.

Conclusions

Over the past decade there have been enormous advances in the understanding of type 2 diabetes and its complications. Although multiple new antihyperglycemic medications have become available, changes frequently are not initiated soon enough, resulting in chronic, poor glycemic control [32]. In order for diabetic patients to achieve glucose goals, treatment must be promptly initiated, carefully monitored and rapidly advanced. If patients are not achieving goals with non-insulin therapy, insulin treatment should be initiated.

References

1   Magee MF, Isley WL; BARI 2D Trial Investigators. Rationale, design, and methods for glycemic control in the Bypass Angioplasty Revascularization Investigation 2 Diabetes (BARI 2D) Trial. Am J Cardiol 2006; 97:20G–30G.
2   Gerstein HC, Riddle MC, Kendall DM, et al; ACCORD Study Group. Glycemia treatment strategies in the Action to Control Cardiovascular Risk in Diabetes (ACCORD) trial. Am J Cardiol 2007; 99:34i-343i.

3   Nathan DM, Buse JB, Davidson MB, et al. Management of hyperglycemia in type 2 diabetes: A consensus algorithm for the initiation and adjustment of therapy: a consensus statement from the American Diabetes Association and the European Association for the Study of Diabetes. Diabetes Care 2006; 29:1963–1972.

4   Bolen S, Feldman L, Vassy J, et al. Systematic review: comparative effectiveness and safety of oral medications for type 2 diabetes mellitus. Ann Intern Med 2007; 147:386–399.

5   Grant RW, Wexler DJ, Watson AJ, et al. How doctors choose medications to treat type 2 diabetes: a national survey of specialists and academic generalists. Diabetes Care 2007; 30:1448–1453.

6   DeFronzo, RA. Lilly lecture 1987. The triumvirate: beta-cell, muscle, liver. A collusion responsible for NIDDM. Diabetes 1988; 37:667–687.

7   Drucker, DJ. The role of gut hormones in glucose homeostasis. J Clin Invest 2007; 117:24–32.

8   Schmitz O, Brock B, Rungby J. Amylin agonists: a novel approach in the treatment of diabetes. Diabetes 2004; 53(Suppl 3):S233-S238.

9   Effect of intensive blood-glucose control with metformin on complications in overweight patients with type 2 diabetes (UKPDS 34). UK Prospective Diabetes Study (UKPDS) Group. Lancet 1998; 352:854–865.

10 DeFronzo RA, Goodman AM. Efficacy of metformin in patients with non-insulin-dependent diabetes mellitus. The Multicenter Metformin Study Group. N Engl J Med 1995; 333:541–549.

11 Goldner MG, Knatterud GL, Prout TE. Effects of hypoglycemic agents on vascular complications in patients with adult-onset diabetes. 3. Clinical implications of UGDP results. JAMA 1971; 218:1400–1410.

12 Intensive blood-glucose control with sulphonylureas or insulin compared with conventional treatment and risk of complications in patients with type 2 diabetes (UKPDS 33). UK Prospective Diabetes Study (UKPDS) Group. Lancet 1998; 352:837–853.

13 Landgraf R, Bilo HJ, Muller PG. A comparison of repaglinide and glibenclamide in the treatment of type 2 diabetic patients previously treated with sulphonylureas. Eur J Clin Pharmacol 1999; 55:165–171.

14 Rosenstock J, Hassman DR, Madder RD, et al. Repaglinide versus nateglinide monotherapy: a randomized, multicenter study. Diabetes Care 2004; 27:1265–1270.

15 Yki-Jarvinen, H. Thiazolidinediones. N Engl J Med 2004; 351:1106–1118.

16 Nissen, SE and Wolski k. Effect of rosiglitazone on the risk of myocardial infarction and death from cardiovascular causes. N Engl J Med 2007; 356:2457–2471.

17 Home PD, Pocock SJ, Beck-Nielsen H, et al; RECORD Study Group. Rosiglitazone evaluated for cardiovascular outcomes--an interim analysis. N Engl J Med 2007; 357:28–38.

18 Dormandy JA, Charbonnel B, Eckland DJ, et al; PROactive investigators. Secondary prevention of macrovascular events in patients with type 2 diabetes in the PROactive Study (PROspective pioglitAzone Clinical Trial In macroVascular Events): a randomised controlled trial. Lancet 2005; 366:1279–1289.

19 Kahn SE, Haffner SM, Heise MA, et al; ADOPT Study Group. Glycemic durability of rosiglitazone, metformin, or glyburide monotherapy. N Engl J Med 2006; 355:2427–2443.

20 http://www.fda.gov/medwatch/safety/2007/safety07.htm#actos. [Last accessed August 1, 2007].

21 Janghorbani M, Van Dam RM, Willett WC, et al. Systematic review of type 1 and type 2 diabetes mellitus and risk of fracture. Am J Epidemiol 2007; 166:495–505.

22 Amori RE, Lau J, Pittas AG. Efficacy and safety of incretin therapy in type 2 diabetes: systematic review and meta-analysis. JAMA 2007; 298:194–206.

23 Holst JJ, Deacon CF. Inhibition of the activity of dipeptidyl-peptidase IV as a treatment for type 2 diabetes. Diabetes 1998; 47:1663-1670.

24 Hollander PA, Levy P, Fineman MS, et al. Pramlintide as an adjunct to insulin therapy improves long-term glycemic and weight control in patients with type 2 diabetes: a 1-year randomized controlled trial. Diabetes Care 2003; 26:784–790.

25 Colagiuri S, Cull CA, Holman RR. Are lower fasting plasma glucose levels at diagnosis of type 2 diabetes associated with improved outcomes?: U.K. Prospective Diabetes Study 61. Diabetes Care 2002; 25:1410–1417.

26 DeFronzo RA, Ratner RE, Han J, et al. Effects of exenatide (exendin-4) on glycemic control and weight over 30 weeks in metformin-treated patients with type 2 diabetes. Diabetes Care 2005; 28:1092-1100.

27 Fonseca V, Rosenstock J, Patwardhan R, et al. Effect of metformin and rosiglitazone combination therapy in patients with type 2 diabetes mellitus: a randomized controlled trial. JAMA 2000; 283:1695–1702.

28 Charbonnel B, Karasik A, Liu J, et al; Sitagliptin Study 020 Group. Efficacy and safety of the dipeptidyl peptidase-4 inhibitor sitagliptin added to ongoing metformin therapy in patients with type 2 diabetes inadequately controlled with metformin alone. Diabetes Care 2006; 29(12):2638–2643.

29 Triplitt C, Glass L, Miyazaki Y, et al. Comparison of glargine insulin versus rosiglitazone addition in poorly controlled type 2 diabetic patients on metformin plus sulfonylurea. Diabetes Care 2006; 29:2371–2377.

30. Heine RJ, Van Gaal LF, Johns D, et al. for the GWAA Study Group. Exenatide versus insulin glargine in patients with suboptimally controlled type 2 diabetes. Ann Intern Med 2005; 143:559–569.

31 Schwartz S, Sievers R, Strange P, et al. INS-2061 Study Team. Insulin 70/30 mix plus metformin versus triple oral therapy in the treatment of type 2 diabetes after failure of two oral drugs: efficacy, safety, and cost analysis. Diabetes Care 2003; 26:2238–2243.

32 Grant RW, Buse JB, Meigs JB. Quality of diabetes care in U.S. academic medical centers: low rates of medical regimen change. Diabetes Care 2005; 28:337–442.

33 AACE Diabetes Mellitus Clinical Practice Guidelines Task Force. American Association of Clinical Endocrinologists medical guidelines for clinical practice for the management of diabetes mellitus. Endocr Pract 2007; 13(Suppl 1):1–68.

Chapter 4

Insulin in the management of type 2 diabetes

Insulin is the most the effective available medication for treating hyperglycemia in type 2 diabetes. If used appropriately, it can decrease any level of elevated A1C to, or close to, the desired goal. This chapter begins with a presentation of indications for insulin therapy in type 2 diabetes. Normal physiological insulin patterns will be reviewed, highlighting how awareness of these patterns can guide the development of insulin treatment regimens. The next section will provide an overview of the characteristics of available insulin preparations. The chapter will end with a discussion of potential strategies for initiating and advancing insulin therapy.

Indications

Whereas insulin therapy is required in all patients with type 1 diabetes, the decision of how and when to start insulin in type 2 diabetes is not as straightforward. Insulin usually should be started immediately in patients with marked weight loss, severe hyperglycemia, or ketosis. In the absence of these features, insulin should be added when glycemic goals are not met with one or more non-insulin agents, or when glycemic goals are unlikely to be achieved with non-insulin therapy [1]. After the glucose is controlled and symptoms are relieved, it may be possible to withdraw the insulin at a later time. Early treatment with insulin may potentially lead to diabetes remissions lasting several years, during which A1C is normal without the need for any medication [2, 3]. It is important to note that, when it is indicated, initiation of insulin therapy should not be delayed. This unnecessarily exposes the patient to the adverse physiological consequences of prolonged hyperglycemia.

Insulin secretion in individuals without diabetes

When considering insulin therapy, it is helpful to keep normal insulin patterns in mind. Euglycemia can best be achieved, and hypoglycemia minimized, by

V.A. Fonseca et al., *Diabetes in Clinical Practice*,
DOI 10.1007/978-1-84882-103-3_4, © Springer-Verlag London Limited 2010

using insulin regimens that supplement insulin in as physiological a way as possible. In patients with normal glucose tolerance, insulin secretion is tightly regulated by the prevailing glucose level (*see* Figure 4.1). Basal insulin, which is secreted even in the absence of nutritional intake, suppresses hepatic glucose production and maintains normoglycemia in the fasting state. In response to a meal, insulin levels rise and fall precisely to the degree needed to maintain the plasma glucose in a very narrow range (~80–140 mg/dL; 4.5–7.8 mmol/L).

Both basal and nutritional insulin requirements vary considerably throughout the day, as well as from day to day. Nutritional insulin requirements vary primarily depending on the quantity, composition, and timing of food. Basal requirements tend to decrease with exercise and increase with stress or illness. Basal insulin requirements also may increase as the result of the "dawn phenomenon", which has been attributed to morning rises in growth hormone and cortisol levels.

Types of insulin

The approximate time of onset, peak activity, and duration of action of the available insulin preparations is shown in *Figures 4.2* and *4.3*. Insulin preparations vary with respect to onset and duration of action, which differ due to modifications to human regular insulin that either slow or hasten the time for it to be absorbed into the bloodstream. Relative to human regular insulin, the rapid-acting analogs (insulin lispro, insulin aspart, and insulin glulisine) have a more rapid onset of action, higher peak serum concentration, and shorter duration of action. Inhaled

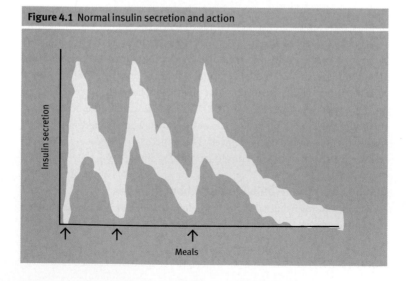

Figure 4.1 Normal insulin secretion and action

Insulin secretion

Meals

Figure 4.2 Profiles of available insulins

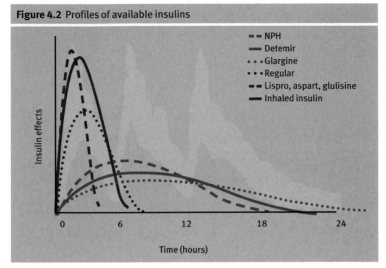

NPH, neutral protamine Hagedorn

human insulin is similar to the rapid-acting analogs in terms of its onset and peak effect. However, its effective duration is slightly longer than the analogs, and comparable to regular insulin. The two basal insulin analogs (insulin glargine and insulin detemir), have a longer duration of action, relative to human basal insulin (neutral protamine Hagedorn or NPH). Premix insulins, which contain fixed amounts of intermediate-acting insulin and short- or rapid-acting insulin, are also available. These mixtures have dual action profiles, consistent with those of the individual components. For example 100 units of 70/30 human insulin have the same effect as 70 units NPH and 30 units regular insulin.

It is important to emphasize that the characteristics outlined in *Figure 4.3* are only approximations. The usually quoted data regarding time of onset and duration of action have not been determined in a standardized fashion. Subcutaneous insulin absorption can be affected by multiple factors including the size of the subcutaneous depot, injection technique, the site of injection, and blood flow. Inhaled insulin has variable absorption characteristics in smokers and in patients with underlying lung disease [4]. In addition, conditions such as impaired renal function can increase the effective duration of action of the administered insulin. Due to these multiple factors, insulin profiles vary significantly from patient to patient. For example, a single daily dose of NPH may be sufficient to last an entire day for one patient, while other patients may require additional injections. Furthermore, variable absorption in the same patient, from day to day, may lead to fluctuations in glycemic control.

Figure 4.3 Approximate duration of action of insulin preparations

Insulin	Onset of action	Peak action	Effective duration
Rapid-acting			
Insulin aspart	5–15 min	30–90 min	<5 h
Insulin lispro	5–15 min	30–90 min	<5 h
Insulin glulisine	5–15 min	30–90 min	<5 h
Insulin inhalation powder	5–15 min	30–90 min	5–8 h
Short-acting			
Regular insulin	30–60 min	2–3 h	5–8 h
Intermediate-acting			
NPH insulin	2–4 h	4–10 h	10–16 h
Long-acting			
Insulin glargine	2–4 h	None	20–24 h
Insulin detemir	3–8 h	None	6–23 h

NPH, neutral protamine Hagedorn. Adapted from reference [5].

Although it has been proposed that pharmacokinetic properties of insulin analogs may translate into improved clinical efficacy, this has not been convincingly demonstrated in clinical trials, especially for type 2 diabetes. Recent meta-analyses of published clinical trials suggest that, compared with human regular insulin, the rapid-acting analogs provide only a small advantage in terms of A1C reductions, and no advantage for hypoglycemia [6–8]. Compared with human NPH insulin, basal analogs (glargine and detemir) have no advantage for A1C and only minor reductions in nocturnal hypoglycemia [8,9]. Detemir insulin has been shown to cause less weight gain than NPH in clinical trials. The mechanism underlying this effect is unclear.

Adverse effects

The two primary adverse effects of insulin therapy in type 2 diabetes are weight gain, which is common, and hypoglycemia, which is uncommon. Insulin is generally associated with a weight gain of about 2–4 kg, which conceivably could have an adverse effect on cardiovascular risk. Insulin detemir has been associated with less or absent weight gain [10–12], and ongoing studies are being done to confirm these observations and to evaluate potential mechanisms. Insulin therapy also is associated with hypoglycemia, although much less frequently than in type 1 diabetes. The frequency of severe hypoglycemia (defined as requiring help from another person to treat) in type 2 diabetes is about the same as in patients treated with SUs (i.e. 0.1 and 0.2 episodes per subject-year) [13].

In contrast to injected insulin, which has essentially no contraindications, multiple safety considerations regarding inhaled insulin have been raised [4]. These include concerns about pulmonary toxicity and an increased risk of hypoglycemia, compared to injected insulin. Inhaled insulin is not recommended for children, pregnant women, patients who have smoked within the past 6 months, and those who have pulmonary disease. Pulmonary testing is required at baseline and after 6 months of treatment. Inhaled insulin was briefly, but is not currently, available in the USA.

General principles of insulin regimens

Initial insulin regimens for patients with type 2 diabetes usually differ considerably from those recommended for type 2 diabetes. Since patients with type 1 diabetes make little or no insulin, treatment is initiated with a goal of mimicking physiological insulin patterns as closely as possible. Effective regimens in type 1 diabetes usually consist of at least one daily injection of basal insulin, in addition to injections of rapid-acting insulin given before each meal. In contrast, since patients with type 2 diabetes usually secrete some endogenous insulin, they frequently can be controlled with only a single injection a day. In later stages of type 2 diabetes, patients may make very little insulin, and thus may require multiple daily injections, similar to the regimens used for type 1 diabetes.

Insulin regimens

The most widely recommended strategy for initiating insulin in type 2 diabetes is to add a single daily injection of basal insulin (NPH, insulin glargine, insulin detemir) to the patient's oral medications. This regimen has been found to be effective in numerous studies [8, 9, 14–22] and controls hyperglycemia in up to 60% of patients [16]. Despite a prevailing misconception that NPH must be given twice a day, it has long been recognized that a single injection of NPH insulin at bedtime yields similar improvements in control as addition of two or more daily injections of insulin [23]. Other possibilities for initial insulin therapy include adding a single injection of glargine [14] or detemir [11] in the morning, or pre-mix insulin at suppertime [24]. Although pre-mix insulin given twice a day [15, 21], or even three times a day [25, 26] has also had good results, these strategies do not appear to be superior to a single injection, and may be less acceptable to patients. If the fasting glucose level is within the target range, but the A1C level remains above goal, additional insulin injections can be added. These are usually given as pre-meal boluses of rapid-acting insulin.

> *Key factor contributing to the success of the regimen*
> This is probably not how the insulin is given, but rather, whether enough insulin is given. For a regimen to be effective, the insulin dose must be increased frequently until targets are achieved.

Relatively large doses of insulin (>1 unit/kg) typically are necessary to overcome the insulin resistance of type 2 diabetes and lower A1C to target levels. Multiple protocols for initiating and increasing insulin have been found to be effective [16, 27]. Furthermore, having patients self-titrate their own doses, according to protocol, appears to be similarly effective as having the insulin adjusted by a healthcare provider [27, 28]. The protocol used in the Treat-To-Target Study [16], which is outlined in *Figure 4.4*, has been widely recommended.

Combination with non-insulin antihyperglycemic agents

Since insulin is usually not a first-line agent in type 2 diabetes, most patients considered for insulin therapy are already taking one or more non-insulin (usually oral) agents. For the majority of patients, insulin does not replace the oral agents; it is typically added to the current regimen. Many effective combinations of insulin and oral agents have been reported [11, 14–17, 19, 22, 24, 29, 30]. When insulin is added to a regimen, continued insulin secretagogue (e.g. SU) treatment provides minimal advantage [19] and probably should be discontinued. The insulin sensitizers, metformin and TZDs, both have been found to be effective in combination with insulin [18, 19, 31]. However, thiazolidinediones should be continued with caution, since combination with insulin may worsen the risk of fluid retention and heart failure.

Figure 4.4 Insulin initiation and titration algorithm

Start with 10 IU/day bedtime basal insulin* and adjust weekly	
Mean of self-monitored FPG values from preceding 2 days	Increase of insulin dosage (IU/day)
≥180 mg/dL (10 mmol/L)	8
140–180 mg/dL (7.8–10.0 mmol/L)	6
120–140 mg/dL (6.7–7.8 mmol/L)	4
100–120 mg/dL (5.6–6.7 mmol/L)	2

* NPH or insulin glargine.
FBG, fasting plasma glucose; NPH, neutral protamine Hagedorn. Adapted from [16].

Figure 4.5 Insulin prefilled delivery device

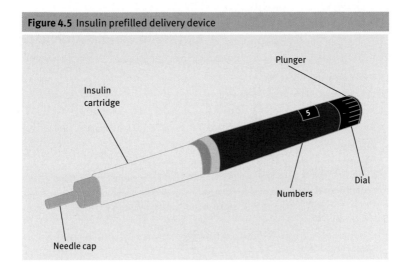

Glucose monitoring

Patient self-monitoring of blood glucose should be individualized, based on the insulin regimen and the patient's symptoms. If a patient is taking only a single bedtime injection of NPH or glargine and does not have symptoms of hypoglycemia, glucose testing once a day in the morning may be sufficient. Patients on multiple daily insulin administrations should test more frequently.

Improving patient adherence

Adherence may be improved if insulin is prescribed in a positive fashion, rather than threatening patients with insulin as a punishment. Patients should be made aware that initiating insulin does not represent a personal failure and that most patients with type 2 diabetes eventually require this treatment due to a decline in endogenous insulin production. Patient preconceptions about use of insulin also need to be addressed [32]. For example, patients frequently believe that once they start on insulin, they will never be able to stop it. They should be reassured it will be possible to withdraw insulin at a later time, particularly if they are able to lose weight and become more physically active. Finally, patients should be educated about the existence of multiple different pre-filled insulin delivery devices (insulin pens), which have been associated with improved satisfaction [33] (*see Figure 4.5*).

Figure 4.6 Potential strategy for insulin initiation and advancement

1 Start 10 units NPH, glargine or detemir at bedtime*

2 Continue metformin. Stop all other antihyperglycemic medications.

3 Have patient check daily FBG

4 Increase insulin doses according to Figure 4.4

5 If A1C meets goal (usually <7%), continue with single daily injection of insulin

6 If A1C is above goal, and FBG has been 100–120 mg/dL for at least 2 months, have patient check BG before breakfast, lunch, dinner, and bedtime

Initiate 1–3 additional insulin injections per day, according to the following:

- if pre-lunch BG is above 180 mg/dL (10 mmol/L), add pre-breakfast insulin aspart, lispro or glulisine
- if pre-dinner BG is above 180 mg/dL (10 mmol/L), add pre-lunch insulin aspart, lispro or glulisine
- if pre-bedtime BG is above 180 mg/dL (10 mmol/L), add pre-dinner insulin aspart, lispro or glulisine

BG, blood glucose; FBG, fasting blood glucose; NPH, neutral protamine Hagedorn.

Conclusion

Many, if not most, patients with type 2 diabetes will eventually require insulin to achieve their glycemic goals. Insulin should be offered to patients as a safe and effective treatment option, not as a punishment. There are multiple ways to give insulin, and the regimen selected probably is not as important as how much insulin is given. Insulin doses must be adjusted frequently until the patient achieves the desired target. One possible strategy for initiating and adjusting insulin is outlined in *Figure 4.6*. Treatment is initiated with a single bedtime injection of basal insulin and the dose is titrated until the fasting glucose is normal. If the fasting glucose normalizes but the A1C remains elevated, additional injections, typically given as pre-meal doses of rapid-acting insulin, may be required. Patients with long-standing diabetes, particularly those who are non-obese, frequently may require multiple daily insulin injections, similar to the regimens used for type 1 diabetes.

References

1   Nathan DM, Buse JB, Davidson MB, et al. Management of hyperglycemia in type 2 diabetes: A consensus algorithm for the initiation and adjustment of therapy: a consensus statement from the American Diabetes Association and the European Association for the Study of Diabetes. Diabetes Care 2006; 29:1963–1972.

2   Ryan EA, Imes S, Wallace C. Short-term intensive insulin therapy in newly diagnosed type 2 diabetes. Diabetes Care 2004; 27:1028–1032.

3   Li Y, Xu W, Liao Z, et al. Induction of long-term glycemic control in newly diagnosed type 2 diabetic patients is associated with improvement of beta-cell function. Diabetes Care. 2004; 27:2597–2602.

4   Ceglia L, Lau J, Pittas AG. Meta-analysis: efficacy and safety of inhaled insulin therapy in adults with diabetes mellitus. Ann Intern Med 2006; 145:665–675.

5   AACE Diabetes Mellitus Clinical Practice Guidelines Task Force. American Association of Clinical Endocrinologists medical guidelines for clinical practice for the management of diabetes mellitus. Endocr Pract 2007; 13(Suppl 1):1-68.

6   Plank J, Siebenhofer A, Berghold A, et al. Systematic review and meta-analysis of short-acting insulin analogues in patients with diabetes mellitus. Arch Intern Med 2005; 165:1337–1344.

7   Siebenhofer A, Plank J, Berghold A, et al. Short acting insulin analogues versus regular human insulin in patients with diabetes mellitus. Cochrane Database Syst Rev 2004(2):CD003287.

8   Gough SC. A review of human and analogue insulin trials. Diabetes Res Clin Pract 2007; 77:1–15.

9   Horvath K, Jeitler K, Berghold A, et al. Long-acting insulin analogues versus NPH insulin (human isophane insulin) for type 2 diabetes mellitus. Cochrane Database Syst Rev 2007(2):CD005613.

10 Meneghini LF, Rosenberg KH, Koenen C, et al. Insulin detemir improves glycaemic control with less hypoglycaemia and no weight gain in patients with type 2 diabetes who were insulin naive or treated with NPH or insulin glargine: clinical practice experience from a German subgroup of the PREDICTIVE study. Diabetes Obes Metab 2007; 9:418–427.

11 Philis-Tsimikas A, Charpentier G, Clauson P, et al. Comparison of once-daily insulin detemir with NPH insulin added to a regimen of oral antidiabetic drugs in poorly controlled type 2 diabetes. Clin Ther 2006; 28:1569–1581.

12 Raslova K, Tamer SC, Clauson P, et al. Insulin detemir results in less weight gain than NPH insulin when used in basal-bolus therapy for type 2 diabetes mellitus, and this advantage increases with baseline body mass index. Clin Drug Investig 2007; 27:279–285.

13 UK Hypoglycaemia Study Group. Risk of hypoglycaemia in types 1 and 2 diabetes: effects of treatment modalities and their duration. Diabetologia 2007; 50:1140–1147.

14 Fritsche A, Schweitzer MA, Häring HU. Glimepiride combined with morning insulin glargine, bedtime neutral protamine hagedorn insulin, or bedtime insulin glargine in patients with type 2 diabetes. A randomized, controlled trial. Ann Intern Med 2003; 138:952–959.

15 Janka HU, Plewe G, Riddle MC, et al. Comparison of basal insulin added to oral agents versus twice-daily premixed insulin as initial insulin therapy for type 2 diabetes. Diabetes Care 2005; 28:254–259.

16 Riddle MC, Rosenstock J, Gerich J; Insulin Glargine 4002 Study Investigators. The treat-to-target trial. randomized addition of glargine or human NPH insulin to oral therapy of type 2 diabetic patients. Diabetes Care 2003; 26:3080–3086.

17 Yki-Jarvinen H. Combination therapies with insulin in type 2 diabetes. Diabetes Care 2001; 24:758–767.

18 Yki-Jarvinen H, Kauppinen-Mäkelin R, Tiikkainen M, et al. Insulin glargine or NPH combined with metformin in type 2 diabetes: the LANMET study. Diabetologia 2006; 49:442–451.

19 Yki-Jarvinen H, Ryysy L, Nikkilä K, et al. Comparison of bedtime insulin regimens in patients with type 2 diabetes mellitus. A randomized, controlled trial. Ann Intern Med 1999; 130:389–396.

20 Cusi K, Cunningham GR, Comstock JP. Safety and efficacy of normalizing fasting glucose with bedtime NPH insulin alone in NIDDM. Diabetes Care 1995; 18:843–851.

21 Raskin P, Allen E, Hollander P, et al; INITIATE Study Group. Initiating insulin therapy in type 2 diabetes: a comparison of biphasic and basal insulin analogs. Diabetes Care 2005; 28:260–265.

22 Heine RJ, Van Gaal LF, Johns D, et al; GWAA Study Group. Exenatide versus insulin glargine in patients with suboptimally controlled type 2 diabetes: a randomized trial. Ann Intern Med 2005; 143:559–569.

23 Yki-Jarvinen H, Kauppila M, Kujansuu E, et al. Comparison of insulin regimens in patients with non-insulin-dependent diabetes mellitus. N Engl J Med 1992; 327:1426–1433.

24 Riddle MC, Schneider J. Beginning insulin treatment of obese patients with evening 70/30 insulin plus glimepiride versus insulin alone. Glimepiride Combination Group. Diabetes Care 1998; 21:1052–1057.

25 Garber AJ, Wahlen J, Wahl T, et al. Attainment of glycaemic goals in type 2 diabetes with once-, twice-, or thrice-daily dosing with biphasic insulin aspart 70/30 (The 1-2-3 study). Diabetes Obes Metab 2006; 8:58–66.

26 Ligthelm RJ, Mouritzen U, Lynggaard H, et al. Biphasic insulin aspart given thrice daily is as efficacious as a basal-bolus insulin regimen with four daily injections: a randomised open-label parallel group four months comparison in patients with type 2 diabetes. Exp Clin Endocrinol Diabetes 2006; 114:511–519.

27 Davies M, Storms F, Shutler S, et al; ATLANTUS Study Group. Improvement of glycemic control in subjects with poorly controlled type 2 diabetes: comparison of two treatment algorithms using insulin glargine. Diabetes Care 2005; 28:1282–1288.

28 Yki-Jarvinen H, Juurinen L, Alvarsson M, et al. Initiate Insulin by Aggressive Titration and Education (INITIATE): a randomized study to compare initiation of insulin combination therapy in type 2 diabetic patients individually and in groups. Diabetes Care 2007; 30:1364–1369.

29 Schwartz S, Sievers R, Strange P, et al; INS-2061 Study Team. Insulin 70/30 mix plus metformin versus triple oral therapy in the treatment of type 2 diabetes after failure of two oral drugs: efficacy, safety, and cost analysis. Diabetes Care 2003; 26:2238–2243.

30 Triplitt C, Glass L, Miyazaki Y, et al. Comparison of glargine insulin versus rosiglitazone addition in poorly controlled type 2 diabetic patients on metformin plus sulfonylurea. Diabetes Care 2006; 29:2371–2377.

31 Strowig SM, Raskin P, Combination therapy using metformin or thiazolidinediones and insulin in the treatment of diabetes mellitus. Diabetes Obes Metab 2005; 7:633–641.

32 Peyrot M, Rubin RR, Lauritzen T, et al. The International DAWN Advisory Panel. Resistance to insulin therapy among patients and providers: results of the cross-national Diabetes Attitudes, Wishes, and Needs (DAWN) study. Diabetes Care 2005; 28:2673–2679.

33 Rubin RR, Peyrot M. Quality of life, treatment satisfaction, and treatment preference associated with use of a pen device delivering a premixed 70/30 insulin aspart suspension (aspart protamine suspension/soluble aspart) versus alternative treatment strategies. Diabetes Care 2004; 27:2495–2497.

34 Freemantle N, Blonde L, Duhot D, et al. Availability of inhaled insulin promotes greater perceived acceptance of insulin therapy in patients with type 2 diabetes. Diabetes Care 2005; 28:427–428.

Chapter 5

Complications of diabetes

Microvascular complications

Microvascular complications are specific for diabetes and are almost certainly related to hyperglycemia (*see Figure 5.1*). Hyperglycemia leads to multiple biochemical changes, some of which are listed in *Figure 5.2*, that cause tissue damage [1, 2]. These lead to changes in various organs as summarized in *Figure 5.1*. Most of these changes can be prevented by good glycemic control which prevents the development of the complications and slows their progression [3].

Eye: Diabetic retinopathy is a specific abnormality: cataract and glaucoma are common.

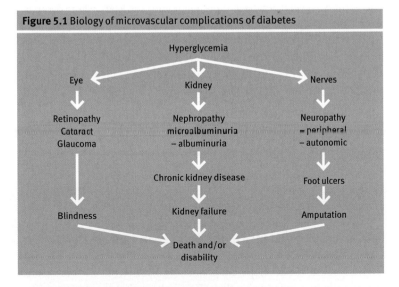

Figure 5.1 Biology of microvascular complications of diabetes

V.A. Fonseca et al., *Diabetes in Clinical Practice*,
DOI 10.1007/978-1-84882-103-3_5, © Springer-Verlag London Limited 2010

Figure 5.2 Mechanisms of diabetes complications

Glycation of proteins (e.g. hemoglobin, collagen, advanced glycation products)

Accumulation of sorbitol and fructose (e.g. in nerves, lens)

Altered protein function and turnover

Cytokine activation and inflammation

Osmotic effects

Activation of protein kinase C

Oxidative stress

Acute changes in nerve conduction velocity

Changes in glomerular filtration rate and renal plasma flow

Kidney: Diabetic nephropathy going through various stages of microalbuminuria to overt proteinuria and kidney failure are specific to diabetes, but other conditions, such as urinary tract infections, may be more common in patients with uncontrolled diabetes.

Nerves: Diabetic neuropathy is specific for diabetes and frequently leads to both peripheral and autonomic neuropathy, and ultimately amputation.

Macrovascular complications

These involve several organs, but predominantly the heart, where coronary artery disease is very common and is associated with decreased morbidity and mortality. Diabetes has been called a cardiovascular risk equivalent due to increased risk of heart disease, even in patients without known prior cardiovascular disease. In addition, congestive heart failure is much more common in patients with diabetes and of greater severity.

Brain: Several vascular diseases, including transient ischemic attack, stroke, and cognitive impairment, have also been described with greater frequency in patients with diabetes.

Extremities: Peripheral vascular disease is also of increased severity, leading to a higher rate of ulceration, gangrene, and amputation.

Role of insulin resistance in the pathogenesis of atherosclerosis

Visceral obesity leads to insulin resistance and increase in free fatty acids. This progresses on to the development of not only diabetes, but other associated factors, including dyslipidemia (low HDL cholesterol, elevated triglycerides, and an increase in small density LDL particles), hypertension, impaired clot

COMPLICATIONS OF DIABETES • 43

breakdown (manifested as an elevation in plasminogen activator inhibitor-1 [PAI-1]), enhanced platelet aggregation, endothelial dysfunction, inflammation, and microalbuminuria (*see Figure 5.3*) [4].

Impact of tight metabolic control on complications
Figure 5.4 summarizes the major clinical trials [6, 8, 9] that have demonstrated that improving control reduces microvascular complications.

Treatment goals to prevent diabetes complications
Figure 5.5 summarizes the risk reduction of various treatments for blood pressure, lipids, and glucose on microvascular and macrovascular events.

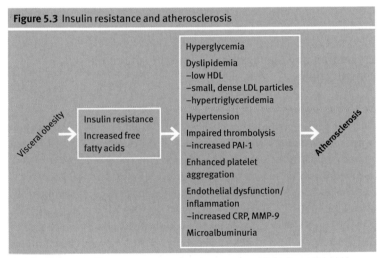

Figure 5.3 Insulin resistance and atherosclerosis

CRP, C reactive protein; HDL, high-density lipoprotein; LDL, low density lipoprotein; MMP-9, matrix metalloproteinase 9; PAI-1, plasminogen activator inhibitor-1.

Figure 5.4 Lowering A1C reduces complications in type 1 and type 2 diabetes

	DCCT	Kumamoto	UKPDS
A1C reduction	9% to 7%	9% to 7%	8% to 7%
Retinopathy ↓	76%	69%	17–21%
Neuropathy ↓	50%	Significantly improved	–
Macrovascular disease ↓	41%	–	16%

DCCT, Diabetes Control and Complications Trial; UKPDS, UK Prospective Diabetes Study. Data from [5–7].

Figure 5.5 Risk reduction with treatment of diabetes

	Microvascular events	Macrovascular events
Blood pressure treatment	20–40%	20–50%
Lipid treatment	–	25–55%
Glucose treatment	12–35%*	10–20%*

*Per 1% A1C reduction.

In this chapter we discuss strategies to detect complications early and treat them or their symptoms early in order to slow their progression and/ or improve the quality of life of the patient. Most of these recommendations are consistent with the standards of care of the American Diabetes Association and other organizations and most are based on evidence from clinical trials [10].

Prevention and management of specific diabetes complications

Nephropathy screening and treatment

Diabetic nephropathy occurs in almost 40% of patients with diabetes and is the single leading cause of end-stage renal disease (ESRD). Persistent albuminuria in the range of 30–299 mg/24 h (microalbuminuria) has been shown to be the earliest stage of diabetic nephropathy in type 1 diabetes and a marker for development of nephropathy in type 2 diabetes. Microalbuminuria is also a well-established marker of increased CVD risk [11, 12]. Patients with microalbuminuria who progress to macroalbuminuria (>300 mg/24 h) are likely to progress to ESRD. Several interventions have been demonstrated to reduce the risk and slow the progression of renal disease.

Intensive diabetes and blood pressure management has been shown in large prospective randomized studies to delay the onset of microalbuminuria and the progression of micro- to macroalbuminuria in patients with type 1 and type 2 diabetes. In addition, angiotensin-converting enzyme (ACE) inhibitors have been shown to reduce severe CVD (i.e. myocardial infarction, stroke, death), thus further supporting the use of these agents in patients with microalbuminuria. Angiotensin receptor blockers (ARBs) have also been shown to reduce the rate of progression from micro- to macroalbuminuria as well as ESRD in patients with type 2 diabetes [13].

Key points: diabetic nephropathy
- Optimize glucose control
- Optimize blood pressure control
- Limit protein intake to the recommended daily allowance (0.8 g/kg) in those with chronic kidney disease
- Test for microalbuminuria annually in type 1 diabetes of ≥5 years duration and in all type 2 patients, starting at diagnosis
- Measure serum creatinine at least annually and estimate glomerular filtration rate (GFR) in all adults with diabetes and stage the level of CKD (*see* Figure 5.6)
- Treat micro- and macroalbuminuria with either ACE inhibitors or ARBs (except during pregnancy)

In patients with type 1 diabetes, with hypertension and any degree of albuminuria, ACE inhibitors have been shown to delay the progression of nephropathy. In patients with type 2 diabetes, hypertension, and microalbuminuria, ACE inhibitors and ARBs have been shown to delay the progression to macroalbuminuria. In patients with type 2 diabetes, hypertension, macroalbuminuria, and renal insufficiency (serum creatinine >1.5 mg/dL, 130 μmol/L), ARBs have been shown to delay the progression of nephropathy. Although ACE inhibitors have not been shown to have this effect (and do not have FDA approval for this indication) their mechanism of action suggests that such an improvement in outcome is likely. In patients unable to tolerate ACE inhibitors and/or ARBs, the use of any antihypertensive agent is appropriate, such as non-dihydropyridine calcium-channel blockers, and beta-blockers, or diuretics for the management of blood pressure. Monitoring of serum potassium levels, for the development of hyperkalemia, and microalbuminuria/proteinuria to assess both response to therapy and progression of disease, are recommended.

Figure 5.6 Stages of chronic kidney disease

Stage	Description	GFR (mL/min/1.73 m² body surface area)
1	Kidney damage with normal or increased GFR	>90
2	Kidney damage with mildly decreased GFR	60–89
3	Moderately decreased GFR	30–59
4	Severely decreased GFR	15–29
5	Kidney failure	<15 or dialysis

GFR, glomerular filtration rate.

Screening for microalbuminuria is best performed by measurement of the albumin-to-creatinine ratio in a random spot collection (*see* Figure 5.7).

Serum creatinine should be measured at least annually for the estimation of GFR in all adults with diabetes regardless of the degree of urine albumin excretion. Serum creatinine alone should be used to estimate GFR and stage the level of CKD (*see* Figure 5.6). The GFR can be easily estimated using a formula such as the Cockroft–Gault formula or a formula developed by Levy et al. [14] using data collected from the Modification of Diet and Renal Disease study. The estimated GFR can easily be calculated by using tools such as the calculator at www.kidney.org/professionals/kdoqi/gfr_calculator. cfm.

Exercise within 24 h, infection, fever, congestive heart failure (CHF), marked hyperglycemia, and hypertension are frequent confounders in screening.

Retinopathy screening and treatment

Diabetic retinopathy is estimated to be the most frequent cause of new cases of blindness among adults aged 20–74 years. Glaucoma, cataracts, and other disorders of the eye also occur earlier and more frequently in people with diabetes.

Intensive diabetes management with the goal of achieving near nor-moglycemia prevents/delays the onset of diabetic retinopathy [3, 8, 15]. In addition to glycemic control, several other factors seem to increase the risk of retinopathy. High blood pressure is a risk factor for the development of macular edema and is associated with the presence of proliferative diabetic retinopathy (PDR). Studies have shown a reduction in the risk of retinopathy with good blood pressure control.

Examinations also can be done using retinal photographs (with or without dilation of the pupil) and having these read by experienced experts in this field. In older-onset patients with severe non-proliferative diabetic

Figure 5.7 Definitions of abnormalities in albumin excretion

Category	Albumin in **spot collection (μg/mg creatine)**
Normal	<30
Microalbuminuria	30–299
Macroalbuminuria (clinical)	≥300

retinopathy (NPDR) or less-than-high-risk PDR, the risk of severe visual loss and vitrectomy is reduced by laser photocoagulation.

Key points in reducing the progression of retinopathy
- Optimal glucose and blood pressure control can substantially reduce the risk and progression of diabetic retinopathy.
- Adults and adolescents with type 1 diabetes: comprehensive eye examination by an ophthalmologist or optometrist within 3–5 years after the onset of diabetes.
- Type 2 diabetes: comprehensive eye examination by an ophthalmologist or optometrist shortly after the diagnosis of diabetes.
- Subsequent examinations should be repeated annually by an ophthalmologist or optometrist.
- Pregnancy: women who are planning pregnancy or who have become pregnant should have a comprehensive eye examination and should be counseled on the risk of development and/or progression of diabetic retinopathy. Eye examination should occur in the first trimester with close follow-up throughout pregnancy and for 1 year postpartum.
- Laser therapy can reduce the risk of vision loss in patients with high-risk characteristics.

Laser photocoagulation surgery is beneficial in reducing the risk of further visual loss, but generally not beneficial in reversing already diminished acuity.

Diabetic neuropathy

The term diabetic neuropathy encompasses a wide range of conditions with diverse clinical manifestations (*see* Figures 5.8 and 5.9). The most common clinical presentation is with chronic sensorimotor DPN and autonomic neuropathy. Although DPN is a diagnosis of exclusion, complex investigations to exclude other conditions are rarely needed.

Patients with diabetes should be screened annually for DPN using tests such as pinprick sensation, temperature and vibration perception (using a 128 Hz tuning fork), 10 g monofilament pressure sensation at the dorsal surface of both great toes, just proximal to the nail bed, and ankle reflexes (*see* Figure 5.10). Combinations of more than one test have >87% sensitivity in detecting DPN. Loss of 10 g monofilament perception and reduced vibration perception predict foot ulcers. A minimum of one clinical test should be carried out annually.

Figure 5.8 Pathophysiology of diabetic neuropathy

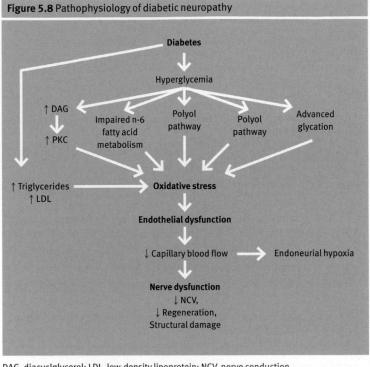

DAG, diacyclglycerol; LDL, low-density lipoprotein; NCV, nerve conduction velocity; PKC, protein kinase C.

Key points: distal symmetric polyneuropathy

- All patients should be screened for distal symmetric polyneuropathy (DPN) at diagnosis and at least annually thereafter, using simple clinical tests. Electrophysiological testing is rarely ever needed.
- Once the diagnosis of DPN is established, special foot care is appropriate for insensate feet to decrease the risk of amputation.
- Simple inspection of insensate feet should be performed at 3- to 6-month intervals. An abnormality should trigger referral for special footwear, preventive specialist, or podiatric care.
- Education of patients about self-care of the feet and referral for special shoes/inserts are vital components of patient management.
- Medications for the relief of specific symptoms related to autonomic neuropathy are recommended.

Figure 5.9 Symptoms of diabetic peripheral nephropathy

Typical neuropathic symptoms

Positive	Negative
Burning pain	Asleep
Knife-like	'Dead'
Electrical sensations	Numbness
Squeezing	Tingling
Constricting	Prickling
Freezing	
Throbbing	
Allodynia	

Negative symptoms are often perceived as unimportant

Symptoms may occur intermittently

Peripheral and symmetric stocking glove distribution

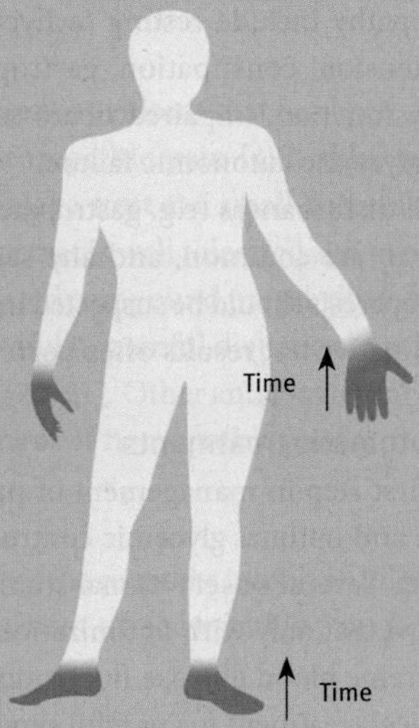

Time

Time

Symptoms and signs progress from distal to proximal over time

Figure 5.10 Assessment of chronic sensorimotor diabetic neuropathy

Annual examination of sensory function in feet and ankle reflexes

Assessment of sensory function with one or more tests
• Pinprick
• Temperature
• Vibration perception (128 Hz tuning fork)
• Pressure sensation (10 g monofilament)

History of neuropathic symptoms

Visual inspection

• Calluses
• Deformities
• Ulcers

Patients with diabetic neuropathy need foot care education and consideration for podiatric referral

Figure 5.12 Conditions associated with increased risk of amputation

- Peripheral neuropathy with loss of protective sensation
- Diabetes >10 years, poor glucose control, presence of other diabetes complications
- Altered biomechanics (in the presence of neuropathy)
- Evidence of increased pressure (erythema, hemorrhage under a callus)
- Bony deformity
- Peripheral vascular disease (decreased or absent pedal pulses)
- A history of ulcers or amputation
- Severe nail pathology

People with neuropathy should have a visual inspection of their feet at every visit with a healthcare professional. Evaluation of neurological status in the low-risk foot should include a quantitative somatosensory threshold test, using the Semmes-Weinstein 5.07 (10 g) monofilament.

People with neuropathy or evidence of increased plantar pressure may be adequately managed with well-fitted walking shoes or athletic shoes. Patients should be educated on the implications of sensory loss. People with evidence of increased plantar pressure (e.g. erythema, warmth, callus, or measured pressure) should use footwear that cushions and redistributes the pressure. Callus can be debrided with a scalpel by a foot care specialist or other health professional with experience and training in foot care. People with bony deformities (e.g. hammer toes, prominent metatarsal heads, or bunions) may need extra-wide shoes or depth shoes. People with extreme bony deformities (e.g. Charcot foot) that cannot be accommodated with commercial therapeutic footwear may need custom-molded shoes.

Initial screening for PAD should include a history for claudication and an assessment of the pedal pulses. Consider measuring the ankle-brachial pressure index (ABI), as many patients with PAD are asymptomatic. Refer patients with significant or a positive ABI for an arterial Doppler study.

Cardiovascular disease

CVD is the major cause of mortality for individuals with diabetes. It is also a major contributor to morbidity and direct and indirect costs of diabetes. Type 2 diabetes is an independent risk factor for macrovascular disease, and its common coexisting conditions (i.e. hypertension and dyslipidemia) are also risk factors.

Studies have shown the efficacy of reducing cardiovascular risk factors in preventing or slowing CVD. The America Diabetes Association/American

College of Cardiology have emphazised the need of controlling the ABCs of diabetes: A1C and aspirin, blood pressure and cholesterol [23].

Hypertension/blood pressure control

Hypertension is a common comorbidity found in the majority of patients with diabetes, particularly those with type 2. Additional risk factors include age, obesity, and ethnicity. Hypertension is a major risk factor for CVD and microvascular complications such as retinopathy and nephropathy.

Key recommendations: monitoring and preventing hypertension
- Blood pressure should be measured at every routine diabetes visit.
- Patients with diabetes should be treated to a systolic blood pressure <130 mmHg and a diastolic blood pressure <80 mmHg. Multiple drug therapy is generally required to achieve blood pressure targets.
- Initial drug therapy for raised blood pressure should be with a drug class demonstrated to reduce CVD events in patients with diabetes (ACE inhibitors, ARBs, beta-blockers, diuretics, and calcium-channel blockers).
- All patients with diabetes and hypertension should be treated with a regimen that includes either an ACE inhibitor or an ARB.
- In patients with type 1 diabetes, with hypertension and any degree of albuminuria, ACE inhibitors have been shown to delay the progression of nephropathy.
- In patients with type 2 diabetes and microalbuminuria, ACE inhibitors and ARBs have been shown to delay the progression to macroalbuminuria.
- In patients with type 2 diabetes and renal insufficiency, ARBs have been shown to delay the progression of nephropathy.

Lowering of blood pressure with regimens based on antihypertensive drugs, including ACE inhibitors, ARBs, beta-blockers, diuretics, and calcium-channel blockers, has been shown to be effective in lowering cardiovascular events. Several studies suggest that ACE inhibitors may be superior to dihydropyridine calcium channel blockers (DCCBs) in reducing cardiovascular events. Additionally, in people with diabetic nephropathy it has been indicated that ARBs may be superior to DCCBs for reducing heart failure but not overall cardiovascular events.

ACE inhibitors have been shown to improve cardiovascular outcomes in patients at high risk for CVD with or without hypertension. In patients

with CHF, the addition of ARBs to either ACE inhibitors or other therapies reduces the risk of cardiovascular death or hospitalization for heart
failure. However, the Antihypertensive and Lipid-Lowering Treatment to
Prevent Heart Attack Trial (ALLHAT), a large randomized trial of different initial blood pressure pharmacological therapies, found no large
differences between initial therapy with a chlorthalidone, amlodipine and
lisinopril [24].

During pregnancy, treatment with ACE inhibitors and ARBs is contrain-
dicated since they are likely to cause fetal damage. Antihypertensive drugs
known to be effective and safe in pregnancy include methyldopa, labetalol,
diltiazem, clonidine, and prazosin. Chronic diuretic use during pregnancy
has been associated with restricted maternal plasma volume, which might
reduce uteroplacental perfusion.

Lipids

Key points in monitoring lipid levels
- In adults, test for lipid disorders at least annually and more often if
  needed to achieve goals. Lifestyle modification including reduction
  of saturated fat and cholesterol intake, weight loss (if indicated), and
  increased physical activity improve the lipid profile.
- In individuals without overt CVD, the primary goal is an LDL <100 mg/
  dL (2.6 mmol/L). In those with overt CVD, the goal is <70 mg/dL
  (1.8 mmol/L).
- For those over the age of 40 years, statin therapy to achieve an LDL reduction of 30–40% regardless of baseline LDL levels is recommended.
- Lower triglycerides to <150 mg/dL (1.7 mmol/L) and raise HDL cholesterol to >40 mg/dL (1.1 mmol/L). In women, an HDL goal 10 mg/
  dL (0.25 mmol/L) higher (>50 mg/dL (1.30 mmol/dL)) should be
  considered.
- Combination therapy using statins and other lipid-lowering agents
  may be necessary to achieve lipid targets but has not been evaluated
  in outcomes studies for either CVD event reduction or safety.

Patients with type 2 diabetes have an increased prevalence of lipid abnormalities that contributes to higher rates of CVD. Lipid management aimed at
lowering LDL cholesterol, raising HDL cholesterol, and lowering triglycerides
has been shown to reduce macrovascular disease and mortality in patients
with type 2 diabetes, particularly in those who have had prior cardiovascular events. In studies using hydroxymethylglutaryl (HMG)-CoA reductase

inhibitors (statins), patients with diabetes achieved significant reductions in coronary and cerebrovascular events . The fibric acid derivative gemfibrozil reductions also leads to reductions in cardiovascular end points [25].

Lifestyle intervention, including medical nutrition therapy (MNT), increased physical activity, weight loss, and smoking cessation, should allow some patients to reach these lipid levels.

Glycemic control can also beneficially modify plasma lipid levels, particularly in patients with very high triglycerides and poor glycemic control.

It is important to note that clinical trials with fibrates and niacin have demonstrated benefits in patients who were not on treatment with statins and that there are no data available on reduction of events with such combinations. The risks may be greater in patients who are treated with combinations of these drugs with high doses of statins.

Additional strategies to decrease CVD are shown in *Figure 5.13*.

Screening for coronary heart disease

To identify the presence of CHD in patients with diabetes without clear or suggestive symptoms of coronary artery disease (CAD), a risk factor-based

Figure 5.13 Additional approaches to decrease CVD events

Antiplatelet agents

Use aspirin therapy (75–162 mg/day) as a secondary prevention strategy in those with diabetes with a history of CVD.

Use aspirin therapy (75–162 mg/day) as a primary prevention strategy

Combination therapy using other antiplatelet agents such as clopidogrel in addition to aspirin should be used in patients with severe and progressive CVD.

Smoking cessation

Advise all patients not to smoke.

Include smoking cessation counseling and other forms of treatment as a routine component of diabetes care.

Other treatments

ACE inhibitors even in the absence of hypertension or albuminuria (in patients >55 years old)
Beta-blockers for patients with CHD (watch for masking of hypoglycemia symptoms)
TZDs are associated with fluid retention and their use can be complicated by the development of CHF. Caution is required in prescribing TZDs in the setting of known CHF or other heart diseases, as well as in patients with preexisting edema or concurrent insulin therapy.

CHD, coronary heart disease; CHF, congestive heart failure; CVD, cardiovascular disease; TZDs, thiazolidinediones.

approach to the initial diagnostic evaluation and subsequent follow-up is recommended (*see* Diabetes PhD at www.diabetes.org or use Framingham score or UK Prospective Diabetes Study Group risk engine).

A diagnostic cardiac stress test should be done in patients with 1) typical or atypical cardiac symptoms and 2) an abnormal resting electrocardiogram (ECG). The screening of asymptomatic patients remains controversial and a significant proportion of patients may have abnormalities, but the significance of this is not clear [26].

A screening cardiac stress test may be considered (but is not essential) in those with 1) a history of peripheral or carotid occlusive disease and 2) sedentary lifestyle, age >35 years, and plans to begin a vigorous exercise program.

Patients with abnormal exercise ECG and patients unable to perform an exercise ECG require additional or alternative testing. Currently, stress nuclear perfusion and stress echocardiography are valuable next-level diagnostic procedures.

Considerations in the patient with multiple complications include:

- Multiple drugs are often needed.
- Renal impairment affects drug use and doses and pharmacokinetics – use more short acting insulin.
- Drug interactions, for example, fludrocortisone for hypotension may increase edema; PDE5 inhibitors interact with nitrates.

References

1 Brownlee M. Biochemistry and molecular cell biology of diabetic complications. Nature 2001; 414:813–820.

2 King GL, Brownlee M. The cellular and molecular mechanisms of diabetic complications. Endocrinol Metab Clin North Am 1996; 25:255–270.

3 Vasudevan AR, Burns A, Fonseca VA. The effectiveness of intensive glycemic control for the prevention of vascular complications in diabetes mellitus. Treat Endocrinol 2006; 5:273–286.

4 Fonseca V, Desouza C, Asnani S, Jialal I. Nontraditional risk factors for cardiovascular disease in diabetes. Endocr Rev 2004; 25:153–175.

5 The effect of intensive treatment of diabetes on the development and progression of long-term complications in insulin-dependent diabetes mellitus. The Diabetes Control and Complications Trial Research Group. N Engl J Med 1993; 329:977–986.

6 Ohkubo Y, Kishikawa H, Araki E, et al. Intensive insulin therapy prevents the progression of diabetic microvascular complications in Japanese patients with non-insulin-dependent diabetes mellitus - a randomized prospective 6-year study. Diabetes Res Clin Pract 1995; 28:103–117.

7 UK Prospective Diabetes Study Group. Tight blood pressure control and risk of macrovascular and microvascular complications in type 2 diabetes: UKPDS 38. BMJ 1998; 317:703–713.

8 The Writing Team for the Diabetes Control and Complications Trial/Epidemiology of Diabetes Interventions and Complications Research Group. Effect of intensive therapy on the microvascular complications of type 1 diabetes mellitus. JAMA 2002; 287:2563–2569.

9 Intensive blood-glucose control with sulphonylureas or insulin compared with conventional treatment and risk of complications in patients with type 2 diabetes (UKPDS 33). UK Prospective Diabetes Study (UKPDS) group. Lancet 1998; 352(9131):837–853.

10 American Diabetes Association. Standards of medical care in diabetes – 2007. Diabetes Care 2007; Jan 30(Suppl 1):S4–S41.

11 Borch-Johnsen K,. Feldt-Rasmussen B, Strandgaard S, Schroll M, Jensen IS. Urinary albumin excretion: an independent predictor of ischemic heart disease. Arterioscler Thromb Vasc Biol 1999; 19:19920–1997.

12 Romundstad S, Holmen J, Kvenild K, Hallan H, Ellekjaer H. Microalbmninuria and all-cause mortality in 2,089 apparently healthy individuals: A 4.4-year follow-up study. The Nordtrondelag Health Study (HUNT), Norway. Am J Kidney Dis 2003; 4:466–473.

13 Scheen AJ. Prevention of type 2 diabetes mellitus through inhibition of the renin-angiotensin system. Drugs 2004; 64:2537–2565.

14 Levey AS, Bosch JP, Lewis JB, et al. A more accurate method to estimate glomerular filtration rate from serum creatinine: a new prediction equation. Modification of Diet in Renal Disease Study Group. Ann Intern Med 1999; 130:461–470.

15 Jawa A Kcomt J, Fonseca VA. Diabetic nephropathy and retinopathy. Med Clin North Am 2004; 88:1001, 36,. xi.

16 Joss JD. Tricyclic antidepressant use in diabetic neuropathy. Ann Pharmacother 1999; 33:996–1000.

17 Max MB, Lynch SA, Muir J, et al. Effects of desipramine, amitriptyline, and fluoxetine on pain in diabetic neuropathy. N Engl J Med 1992; 326:1250–1256.

18 McQuay HJ, Tramèr M, Nye BA, et al. A systematic review of antidepressants in neuropathic pain. Pain 1996; 68:217–227.

19 Backonja M, Beydoun A, Edwards KR, et al. Gabapentin for the symptomatic treatment of painful neuropathy in patients with diabetes mellitus: a randomized controlled trial. JAMA 1998; 280:1831–1836.

20 Rosenstock J, Tuchman M, LaMoreaux L, et al. Pregabalin for the treatment of painful diabetic peripheral neuropathy: a double-blind, placebo-controlled trial. Pain 2004; 110:628–638.

21 Richter RW, Portenoy R, Sharma U, et al. Relief of painful diabetic peripheral neuropathy with pregabalin: a randomized, placebo-controlled trial. J Pain 2005; 6:253–260.

22 Goldstein DJ, Lu Y, Detke MJ, et al. Duloxetine vs. placebo in patients with painful diabetic neuropathy. Pain 2005; 116:109–118.

23 Fight against diabetes and heart disease link intensifies: more efforts needed to help people with diabetes manage the "abcs of diabetes". Available at: http://diabetes.org/for-media/2004-press-releases/fight-diabetes.jsp. Last accessed September 2007.

24 The ALLHAT Officers and Coordinators for the ALLHAT Collaborative Research Group. Major outcomes in high risk hypertensive patients randomized to angiotensin converting enzyme inhibitor or calcium channel blocker vs diuretic. The Antihypertensive and Lipid-Lowering Treatment to Prevent Heart Attack Trial (ALLHAT). JAMA 2002; 288:1981–1997.

25 Boden WE. High-density lipoprotein cholesterol as an independent risk factor in cardiovascular disease: assessing the data from Framingham to the Veterans Affairs High--Density Lipoprotein Intervention Trial. Am J Cardiol 2000; 86:19L–22L.

26 Wackers FJ, Young LH, Inzucchi SE, et al. Detection of silent myocardial ischemia in asymptomatic diabetic subjects: the DIAD study. Diabetes Care 2004; 27:1954–1961.

Chapter 6

Diabetic emergencies

The major diabetic emergencies are:
- diabetic ketoacidosis (DKA)
- hyperosmolar hyperglycemic syndrome (HHS)
- severe hypoglycemia.

All these conditions are associated with significant morbidity and mortality particularly if not managed well. In particular, the mortality rate in HHS still remains high, especially in elderly patients, in whom the condition is more common.

Hyperglycemic crisis

It is important to recognize the underlying precipitating factors in the development of severe hyperglycemia, because their treatment may be critical to recovery.

The most common precipitating factor in the development of DKA or HHS is infection. Other precipitating factors include cerebrovascular accident, alcohol abuse, pancreatitis, myocardial infarction, trauma, and drugs (steroids, antipsychotics, thiazide diuretics, etc.). In addition, new-onset type 1 diabetes or discontinuation of or inadequate insulin in established type 1 diabetes commonly leads to the development of DKA, which may be recurrent in some patients with psychologic problems complicated by eating disorders.

The classic clinical picture includes a history of polyuria, polydipsia, weight loss, vomiting, dehydration, weakness, drowsiness, and finally coma. Physical findings may include signs of dehydration, tachycardia, hypotension, alteration in mental status, shock, and ultimately coma. In addition, acidosis in DKA leads to Kussmaul's respiration.

The classic laboratory findings in DKA and HSS are listed in Figure 6.1.

V.A. Fonseca et al., *Diabetes in Clinical Practice*,
DOI 10.1007/978-1-84882-103-3_6, © Springer-Verlag London Limited 2010

Key laboratory evaluations in hyperglycemic crisis
- Plasma glucose, blood urea nitrogen/creatinine, serum ketones, electrolytes (with calculated anion gap), osmolality
- Urinalysis, including ketones
- Arterial blood gases
- Complete blood count with differential
- Electrocardiogram in older patients and those at risk of myocardial infarction
- Bacterial cultures of urine, blood, throat, etc.; give appropriate antibiotics if infection is suspected

Management

The principles of management of DKA and HHS are summarized in the box. A suggested management protocol is summarized in Figures 6.2 and 6.3 [1].

Fluids and electrolytes

Initial fluid therapy is directed toward expansion of the intravascular and extravascular volume and restoration of renal perfusion. In the absence of cardiac compromise, isotonic saline (0.9% NaCl) is infused at a rate of

Figure 6.1 Classic laboratory findings in diabetic ketoacidosis (DKA) and hyperosmolar hyperglycemic syndrome (HSS)

- Elevated blood ketone body concentration
- Leukocytosis proportional to blood concentration of ketone bodies
- Serum sodium concentration is usually reduced
- Serum potassium concentration may be raised
- Increased plasma osmolality – may be calculated by the following formula:

$$2 [Na] + [glucose]/18$$

where [Na] measured in mEq/L (mmol/L) and [glucose] in mg/dL

- Amylase levels are often elevated in patients with DKA; a serum lipase determination may be beneficial in the differential diagnosis of pancreatitis, but lipase could also be raised in DKA
- Abdominal pain and elevation of serum amylase and liver enzymes are noted more commonly in DKA than in HHS
- DKA is characterized by high-anion gap metabolic acidosis, which must be distinguished from other causes, including lactic acidosis, and ingestion of drugs such as salicylate, methanol, ethylene glycol, and paraldehyde

15–20 ml/kg body weight per hour or greater during the first hour (1–1.5 L in the average adult). Subsequent choice for fluid replacement depends on the state of hydration, serum electrolyte levels, and urinary output. If renal function is reasonable, the infusion should include potassium 20–30 mmol/L until the patient is stable and can tolerate oral supplementation. Successful progress with fluid replacement is judged by hydration status and blood pressure, measurement of fluid input/output, and clinical examination.

Key points in the treatment of diabetic ketoacidosis and hyperosmolar hyperglycemic syndrome

- Rapidly correct dehydration – large amounts of fluids are usually needed
- Correct electrolyte imbalances – pay particular attention to avoiding hypokalemia
- Give bicarbonate injections only in extreme acidosis (pH <7.0); bicarbonate usually corrects itself
- Treat hyperglycemia with low-dose insulin infusion
- Identify and treat precipitating factors
- Take general measures for patients with altered mental status. Avoid aspiration in patients who are vomiting
- Phosphate infusions are controversial but may be given for severe hypophosphatemia

---

Insulin

Insulin therapy, correction of acidosis, and volume expansion decrease serum potassium concentration. To prevent hypokalemia, potassium replacement is initiated after serum levels fall below 5.5 mmol/L, assuming the presence of adequate urine output. Generally, 20–30 mmol potassium (two-thirds as chloride and one-third as phosphate) in each liter of infusion fluid is sufficient to maintain a serum potassium concentration within the normal range of 4–5 mmol/L.

An intravenous bolus of regular insulin at 0.15 U/kg body weight, followed by a continuous infusion of regular insulin at a dose of 0. 1 U/kg per h (5–7 U/h in adults), should be administered. The dose of insulin may be adjusted according to the response. When the plasma glucose reaches 250 mg/dL (14 mmol/L) in DKA or 300 mg/dL (16.5 mmol/L) in HHS, it may be possible to decrease the insulin infusion rate to 0.05–0.1 U/kg per h (3–6 U/h), and dextrose (5–10%) may be added to the intravenous fluids. When acidosis in DKA or mental obtundation and hyperosmolarity in HHS are resolved and the patient begins eating, subcutaneous insulin should be started.

Figure 6.2 Protocol for the management of diabetic ketoacidosis (DKA) in adults*

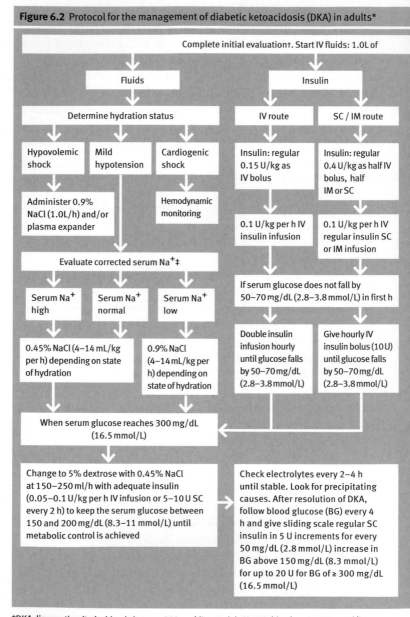

*DKA diagnostic criteria: blood glucose >250 mg/dL, arterial pH <7.3, bicarbonate <15 mmol/L, and moderate ketonuria or ketonemia.

†After history and physical examination, obtain arterial blood gases, complete blood count with differential, urinalysis, blood glucose, blood urea nitrogen, electrolytes, chemistry profile, and creatinine levels, STAT, as well as an electrocardiogram. Obtain chest X-ray and cultures as needed.

Figure 6.2 Continued

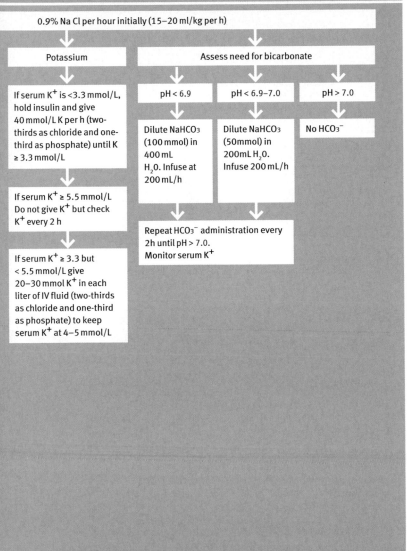

0.9% Na Cl per hour initially (15–20 ml/kg per h)

Potassium

If serum K$^+$ is <3.3 mmol/L, hold insulin and give 40 mmol/L K per h (two-thirds as chloride and one-third as phosphate) until K ≥ 3.3 mmol/L

If serum K$^+$ ≥ 5.5 mmol/L Do not give K$^+$ but check K$^+$ every 2 h

If serum K$^+$ ≥ 3.3 but < 5.5 mmol/L give 20–30 mmol K$^+$ in each liter of IV fluid (two-thirds as chloride and one-third as phosphate) to keep serum K$^+$ at 4–5 mmol/L

Assess need for bicarbonate

pH < 6.9

Dilute NaHCO3 (100 mmol) in 400 mL H$_2$0. Infuse at 200 mL/h

pH < 6.9–7.0

Dilute NaHCO3 (50mmol) in 200mL H$_2$0. Infuse 200 mL/h

pH > 7.0

No HCO3$^-$

Repeat HCO3$^-$ administration every 2h until pH > 7.0. Monitor serum K$^+$

‡Serum Na+ should be corrected for hyperglycemia (for each 100 mg/dL glucose >100 mg/dL (5.5 mmol/L > 5.5 mmol/L), add 1.6 mmol to sodium value for corrected serum sodium value). IM, intramuscular; IV, intravenous; SC, subcutaneous.
Reproduced with permission from Kitabchi et al [1].

Figure 6.3 Protocol for the management of hyperosmolar hyperglycemic

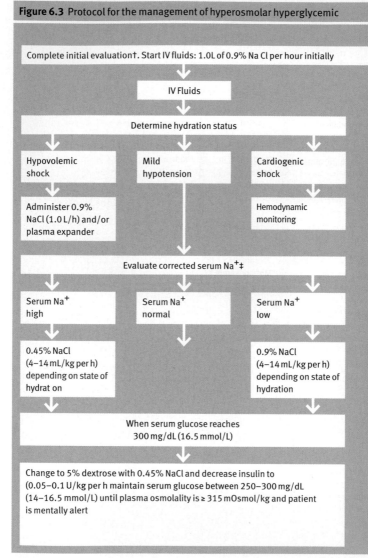

Complete initial evaluation†. Start IV fluids: 1.0L of 0.9% Na Cl per hour initially

IV Fluids

Determine hydration status

Hypovolemic shock

Mild hypotension

Cardiogenic shock

Administer 0.9% NaCl (1.0 L/h) and/or plasma expander

Hemodynamic monitoring

Evaluate corrected serum Na$^+$‡

Serum Na$^+$ high

Serum Na$^+$ normal

Serum Na$^+$ low

0.45% NaCl (4–14 mL/kg per h) depending on state of hydrat on

0.9% NaCl (4–14 mL/kg per h) depending on state of hydration

When serum glucose reaches 300 mg/dL (16.5 mmol/L)

Change to 5% dextrose with 0.45% NaCl and decrease insulin to (0.05–0.1 U/kg per h maintain serum glucose between 250–300 mg/dL (14–16.5 mmol/L) until plasma osmolality is ≥ 315 mOsmol/kg and patient is mentally alert

*Diagnostic criteria: blood glucose >600 mg/dL, arterial pH >7.3, bicarbonate >15 mmol/L, effective serum osmolality >320 mosmol/kg H_2O, and mild ketonuria or ketonemia.

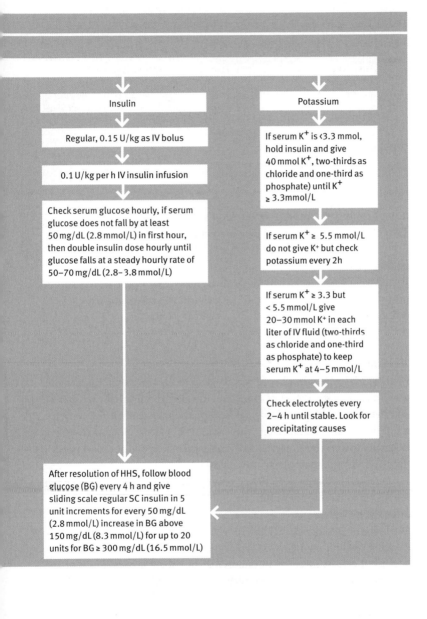

Insulin

Regular, 0.15 U/kg as IV bolus

0.1 U/kg per h IV insulin infusion

Check serum glucose hourly, if serum glucose does not fall by at least 50 mg/dL (2.8 mmol/L) in first hour, then double insulin dose hourly until glucose falls at a steady hourly rate of 50–70 mg/dL (2.8–3.8 mmol/L)

Potassium

If serum K^+ is <3.3 mmol, hold insulin and give 40 mmol K^+, two-thirds as chloride and one-third as phosphate) until K^+ ≥ 3.3mmol/L

If serum K^+ ≥ 5.5 mmol/L do not give K^+ but check potassium every 2h

If serum K^+ ≥ 3.3 but < 5.5 mmol/L give 20–30 mmol K^+ in each liter of IV fluid (two-thirds as chloride and one-third as phosphate) to keep serum K^+ at 4–5 mmol/L

Check electrolytes every 2–4 h until stable. Look for precipitating causes

After resolution of HHS, follow blood glucose (BG) every 4 h and give sliding scale regular SC insulin in 5 unit increments for every 50 mg/dL (2.8 mmol/L) increase in BG above 150 mg/dL (8.3 mmol/L) for up to 20 units for BG ≥ 300 mg/dL (16.5 mmol/L)

Figure 6.4 Complications of diabetic ketoacidosis and their prevention

Complication	Prevention
Hypokalemia	Give K$^+$ even if normal
Hypoglycemia	Avoid excess insulin
Cerebral edema	Gradual replacement of sodium and water deficits in patients who are hyperosmolar (maximal reduction in osmolality 3 mOsmol/kg H$_2$O per h) and the addition of dextrose to the hydrating solution once blood glucose reaches 250 mg/dL (14 mmol/L)
Pulmonary edema	
Aspiration pneumonia	Empty stomach if vomitting

Complications of diabetic ketoacidosis

The complications of DKA and their prevention are summarized in Figure 6.4.

Hypoglycemia

Hypoglycemia is the major limiting factor in intensive treatment with insulin and to a lesser extent with sulfonylureas [2]. It is classified as severe if another person's assistance is needed for treatment. In severe cases hospitalization is needed; if not treated promptly, they can result in injury, seizures, coma, and death.

Treatment

Episodes of asymptomatic hypoglycemia (detected by self-monitoring of blood glucose) and most episodes of symptomatic hypoglycemia can be self-treated effectively by ingestion of glucose tablets or carbohydrate in the form of juice, a soft drink, milk, crackers, or a meal. An initial glucose dose of 15–20 g is essential and sometimes may need to be repeated or followed by a meal, because the glycemic response to oral glucose is usually of short duration.

Parenteral therapy is necessary when a hypoglycemic patient is unable to take carbohydrate orally. Intravenous glucose is the preferable treatment of severe hypoglycemia, if venous access is available. This is usually given as a bolus of 50% dextrose followed by a subsequent glucose infusion, and frequent feeding is often required. Parenteral glucagon is an alternative because it can be given by intramuscular or subcutaneous injection and used by family members to treat severe hypoglycemia the home setting.

References

1   Kitabchi AE, Umpierrez GE, Murphy MB, et al. Management of hyperglycemic crises in patients with diabetes. Diabetes Care 2001; 24:131–53.
2   Cryer PE, Davis SN, Shamoon H. Hypoglycemia in diabetes. Diabetes Care 2003; 26:1902–12.

Chapter 7

Patient education

Goals of patient education

Stated succinctly, the goal of National Standards for Diabetes Self-Management Education (DSME) is to help people cope with the demands of diabetes so that ultimately they can delay or prevent the complications of diabetes. As research in diabetes has progressed, we have learned that complications, once thought a natural progression of the disease, can potentially be delayed and even prevented. Healthcare providers began to consider the various components involved in diabetes disease management which brought into focus the significant role of the diabetes patient in the disease management process (*see* Figure 7.1).

While patients with diabetes provide approximately 95% of all of their care, the self-management regimen required in diabetes may be one of the most difficult of all chronic diseases. Among the challenges are included:

- Monitoring blood glucose levels multiple times daily, an uncomfortable process requiring collection of a blood sample.
- Understanding how to use the result of the blood glucose monitoring effort to assist in management.
- Understanding the nature of diabetes and its complications.
- Observing to identify signs and symptoms of emerging problems.
- Taking medications appropriately, including complex insulin regimens.
- Understanding the roles of the macronutrients and complying with an appropriate meal plan.
- Understanding the role of exercise in diabetes and following an appropriate exercise plan.

The American Diabetes Association developed the National Standards for DSME, which is updated and published annually, to define standards for the provision of reimbursable diabetes self-management education. These

V.A. Fonseca et al., *Diabetes in Clinical Practice*,
DOI 10.1007/978-1-84882-103-3_7, © Springer-Verlag London Limited 2010

Figure 7.1 Diabetes self-management

Assist patients with the following information:

• diabetes disease and its progressive nature

• available treatment options

• details of monitoring for early indications of emergent health problems

• significance of adhering to all self-management procedures

• behavior modifications that will improve overall health

Specific self-management issues to address:

1   Blood glucose monitoring: how-to, frequency, alternate site, recording blood glucose (daily log)

2   Hypoglycemia: symptoms, treatments, prevention

3   Insulin injection devices: all available options

4   Sick-day rules: monitoring frequency with goals, diet options, prevention techniques, when to report blood glucose levels

5   Pre-pregnancy counseling

6   Medications: timing (AM, PM), frequency (once, twice, three times per day), how (with food, empty stomach), cautions (with other meds, alone)

7   Meal planning: (*see* Chapter 4)

8   Exercise: (*see* Chapter 4)

Data in part from [1].

standards include specific content areas to be included in the education process. Required topics include [2]:

• diabetes disease process and treatment options;

• nutrition management;

• physical activity;

• medications use for therapeutic effectiveness;

• blood glucose monitoring;

• preventing, detecting and treating acute complications;

• preventing, detecting and treating chronic complications;

• goal setting to promote health and resolve problems;

• psychosocial adjustment; and

• preconception care: diabetes management during pregnancy and gestational diabetes management.

Diabetes self-management education should be acknowledged by the health-care provider as an integral part of the diabetes treatment plan, recognizing that patient development of necessary problem-solving skills will be based on a thorough knowledge of this complex disease and treatment options [3]. It has been demonstrated that patient self-management of diabetes, including blood glucose monitoring and adjustment of medications, can improve patient outcomes for patients with type 2 diabetes [4]. The DSME program should include instruction on goal-setting strategies that will encourage patients to work with diabetes teams to define treatment goals and choose therapeutic interventions that are acceptable to the patient and will facilitate success [5].

Diabetes self-management education must be individualized for each patient based on personal characteristics, learning studies, and treatment plans [6]. The individual assessment, which is a necessary part of the education process, determines whether the process will meet individual needs; however, group educational processes, as part of the overall diabetes education program, have been demonstrated to be quite effective [7]. *Figure 7.2* highlights the key areas that are important as part of diabetes education.

DSME must strive to provide the necessary information (knowledge, behavior modification, and self-responsibility), in an accessible and acceptable format, to empower people with diabetes to accumulate the knowledge that enables them to successfully self-manage their diabetes, based on their own informed choices. Ultimately this will help patients to attain their self-determined treatment goals.

Monitoring glycemic control (urine/blood glucose, metabolic targets)

Glycemic goals differ slightly based on recommendations by leading authorities; however, there are a variety of other issues to consider when working with patients to set glycemic goals. Since publication of the Diabetes Control and Complications Trial (DCCT), A1C has been recognized as the gold standard for monitoring blood glucose control (*see* Figure 7.3).

However, the limitations of A1C in evaluating blood glucose control must be reviewed. A1C does not provide information representative of the frequent variations in glucose levels daily as related to various times of the day, various

Figure 7.2 Principles of good practice for diabetes education
Education should incorporate principles of adult learning
Education should be provided by a well-trained, multidisciplinary team
Education should take into account culture, ethnicity, disability and other relevant issues
Education should involve a variety of education techniques to promote active learning
Education must empower patients to make knowledgeable choices in their treatment plans, to skillfully manage the requirements of control over diabetes and understand the consequences of their actions

Data from [8, 9].

Figure 7.3 Goals for glycemic control

American Diabetes Association

Hemoglobin A1C	<7%
Preprandial glucose	90–130 mg/dL (5.0–7.2 mmol/L)
Two hour postprandial glucose	<180 mg/dL (<10 mmol/L)

American Association of Clinical Endocrinologists

Hemoglobin A1C	<6.5%
Preprandial glucose	<110 mg/dL
Two-hour postprandial glucose	<140 mg/dL

Data from Diabetes Care 2007; 30 (suppl. 1):S10 and ACE/AACE Diabetes Road Map Task Force. Road maps to achieve glycemic control in type 2 diabetes mellitus. Endocr Pract, 2007; 13(3):261–264.

mealtime or fasting levels, or glucose levels related to activities, stressors of all kinds and/or specific medications. Most of this information must be gathered from self-monitored blood glucose (SMBG) logs [10]. While noninvasive and inexpensive, urine glucose testing only detects glucose levels above the individual's renal threshold, rendering this means of glucose monitoring ineffective for achieving currently accepted levels of glucose control [11].

In a study of 201 insulin-requiring patients with diabetes, intensive self-monitoring of blood glucose demonstrated significant reductions in A1C [12]. Self-monitored blood glucose testing provides educational opportunities for patients, complementing the education process by providing information representative of the impact of multiple variables on glucose levels, including meal planning and/or specific foods, exercise, stress, and medications. However, a recently-completed trial, the Diabetes Glycaemic Education and Monitoring (DiGEM) study, determined that for reasonably well-controlled, non-insulin treated patients there is no adequate evidence that self-monitoring blood glucose improves glycemic control [13]. Nonetheless, substantial evidence exists confirming the value of self-monitoring in insulin-treated patients.

Identifying and overcoming barriers to effective self-care

Patients who have been diagnosed with diabetes are immediately faced with a multitude of challenges, all related to maintaining the quality of their daily life. Research has well demonstrated the galaxy of complications that can follow the onset of diabetes, in the absence of good diabetes management. Yet, good diabetes management requires acquiring numerous skills, making countless lifestyle changes and adjustments, and investing significant amounts of time and effort into a lengthy, complicated education process. Seven specific self-care behaviors have been identified as inherent in good self-care in diabetes (*see* Figure 7.4).

Unfortunately, many patients encounter barriers that prevent them from accomplishing effective self-care (*see* Figure 7.5). Barriers encountered by the healthcare provider that should also be considered are:

- Treatment goals and regimens: consider the patient's overall health and the patient's goals for diabetes treatment once the patient has been educated about diabetes and potential complications. Adjust therapies based on those findings.

Figure 7.4 Seven self-care behaviors

1 Healthy eating
2 Being active
3 Taking medication
4 Monitoring blood glucose
5 Problem-solving
6 Healthy coping
7 Reducing risks

Data from [14].

Figure 7.5 Patient-perceived barriers to effective self-care

1 Frequent lack of symptoms with elevated blood glucose, blood pressure and cholesterol levels – failure to incentivise patients
2 Lack of knowledge and understanding of meal plans
3 Requirements for multiple, daily interventions
4 Lack of individualized, coordinated care
5 Occasions of hypoglycemia that may occur as the appropriate treatment plan is developed and implemented
6 Limited resources
7 Problems related to glucose testing.
8 Inconvenient, expensive group diabetes education programs
9 Inability to cope with appropriate medication treatment regimen as a result of poor information or understanding.
10 Inability or unwillingness to participate in exercise activities
11 Perceived loss of control
12 Psychological impact of chronic disease and related issues

Data from [9, 15–17].

- Management of hypoglycemia: determine that the patient has been educated on both the management of hypoglycemia and the prevention of hypoglycemia. Make incremental changes to therapies frequently until goals have been achieved.
- Clinical inertia: make incremental changes to patient therapies, based on treatment goals. Consider using staff nurse phone visits to receive patient reports of blood glucose logs and to make protocol-driven treatment changes for insulin-treated patients.
- Use of insulin as a treatment option: provide patient with information regarding this option at diagnosis or new patient "first" visit. Current treatment options include various injection devices as well as inhaled insulin therapy.

Healthcare providers can anticipate many of those barriers mentioned in Figure 7.5 and above, and prepare patients to more effectively manage obstacles as they are encountered.

We have acknowledged that patients must be "team leaders" of their diabetes team because of their "expertise" on their own knowledge, beliefs, support system, attitudes, resources, culture, likes and dislikes, habits, etc. Those same factors play a role not only in management of diabetes but in the education process as well. Education that promotes adherence is patient-focused, includes collaboration between healthcare providers and patients, and empowers patients to make positive behavior changes.

Studies indicate that people with diabetes are 1.5 to 2 times more inclined to be clinically depressed than people who do not have diabetes. Further, this depression in the population of people with diabetes increases their risk of mortality by 30%. Depression can be linked to poor self-care, poor diabetes control and higher risks of complications [18, 19].

In a recent study on self-care behaviors in diabetes, it was determined that only 6% of patients performed the four self-care behaviors under study at recommended levels. These included: physical activity, fruits and vegetable consumption, home blood glucose testing and home foot examination. Interestingly, performance of all self-care behaviors was higher in the insulin-requiring patients. Nearly 90% of all patients in the study engaged in at least one self-care behavior but the percentage dropped dramatically as the number of self-care behaviors being observed increased [20]. Another recent study determined that a consistent relationship exists between self-efficacy and self-management in diabetes, identifying self-efficacy as a viable target for educational interventions designed to improve self-care [21]. Diabetes education promotes self-care by providing knowledge; however, knowledge alone will not produce successful self-care. Self-efficacy is an integral

Figure 7.6 Effective strategies for successful diabetes self-management

1	Collaborative relationship with healthcare providers
2	Clearly define "good glycemic control"
3	Positive patient and provider attitudes
4	Ensure adequate monitoring of blood glucose levels
5	Formal/informal support groups
6	Address co-morbidities that are involved in secondary complications
7	Ample resources exist for good self-management
8	Appropriate medication management, including combinations of agents
9	Working with diabetes team in both formal and informal education processes to empower patients for good self-management
10	Healthcare team phone follow-ups

Data from [14, 15, 24, 25].

part of good self-care in diabetes. If people believe they will be successful, they will be motivated to succeed [22]. This is in keeping with the patient empowerment philosophy, as applied in patient-centered practices, involving interactions between healthcare providers and patients that are positive and well-informed [23] (*see* Figure 7.6). These interactions are based on the chronic care model discussed in Chapter 4 [26].

Patient resources

American Association of Diabetes Educators. Available at: www.diabeteseducator. org/. Last accessed September 2007. Diabetes Educator Access Line: 1-800-TEAMUP4 (1-800-832-6874) or 1-800-338-3633.

American Diabetes Association (ADA). Available at: www.diabetes.org. Last accessed September 2007. National Call Center:1-800-DIABETES (1-800-342-2383).

American Dietetic Association (ADA). Available at: www.eatright.org. Last accessed September 2007. Telephone: 1-800-877-1600.

Diabetes Action Research and Education Foundation. Available at: www.diabetesaction.org. Last accessed September 2007. Telephone: 1-202-333-4520.

Diabetes and Me. Available at www.cdc.gov/diabetes/consumer/index.htm. Last accessed September 2007. CDC Diabetes Public Inquiries: 1-800-CDC-INFO.

Diabetes Exercise and Sports Association (DESA). Available at: www.diabetes-exercise.org. Last accessed September 2007. Telephone: 1-800-898-4322.

National Diabetes Education Program. About Diabetes and Pre-diabetes. Available at: http://ndep.nih.gov/diabetes/diabetes.htm. Last accessed September 2007. Telephone: 1-800-438-5383.

National Diabetes Information Clearinghouse (NDIC). Available at: http://diabetes.niddk.nih. gov/. Last accessed September 2007.

National Kidney and Urologic Disease Information Clearinghouse (NKUDIC). Available at: http://kidney.niddk.nih.gov. Last accessed September 2007. Telephone: 1-800-891-5390

Weight-control Information Network (WIN). Available at: http://win.niddk.nih.gov. Last accessed September 2007. Telephone: 1-877-946-4627

References

1 International Diabetes Federation. Diabetes Education: A Right for All. Position Statement. Available at: www.idf.org/home/index.cfm?unode=A1205437-D4F1-40B3-B69D-2E536E0F62CB. Last accessed September 2007.

2 Mensing C, Boucher J, Cypress M, et al. National Standards for Diabetes Self-Management Education. Diabetes Care 2007; 30(Suppl 1):S96–S103.

3 National Institute of health. What we want to achieve through systems changes: patient-centered care: patient education. Available at: www.betterdiabetescare.nih.gov/WHATpatientcenteredcare.htm. Last accessed September 2007.

4 Kronsbein P, Jorgens V, Muhlhauser I, et al. Evaluation of a structured treatment and teaching programme on non-insulin dependent diabetes. Lancet 1988; 2:1407–1411.

5 Berger M, Muhlhauser I. Diabetes care and patient-oriented outcomes. JAMA 1999; 281:1676–1678.

6 American Association of Diabetes Educators. AADE position statement. Individualization of diabetes self-management education. Diabetes Educ 2007; 33:45–49.

7 Piette, JD. The effectiveness of diabetes self-management education: an overview of published studies. Available at: www.eatlas.idf.org/webdata/docs/Effectiveness%20of%20diabetes%20education.pdf. Last accessed September 2007.

8 National Institute for Clinical Excellence. Guidance on the use of patient-education models for diabetes. April 2003. Available at: www.nice.org.uk/pdf/FAD_patient_educationmodels_diabetes.pdf. Last accessed September 2007.

9 Agency for Healthcare Research and Quality. Improving care for diabetes patients through intensive therapy and a team approach. Available at: www.ahrq.gov/research/diabria/diabria.pdf. Last accessed September 2007.

10 Dailey, G. Assessing glycemic control with self-monitoring of blood glucose and hemoglobin A1c measurements. Mayo Clin Proc 2007; 82:229–236.

11 Renard E. Monitoring glycemic control: the importance of self-monitoring of blood glucose. Am J Med 2005; 118:12–19.

12 Murata GH, Adam, KD, Shah JH, et al. Intensified blood glucose monitoring improves glycemic control in stable, insulin-treated veterans with type 2 diabetes. Diabetes Care 2003; 26:1759–1763.

13 Farmer A, Wade A, Goyder E, et al. Impact of self monitoring of blood glucose in the management of patients with non-insulin treated diabetes: open parallel group randomized trial. BMJ 2007; 335:132.

14 Austin MM. Importance of self-care behaviors in diabetes management. US Endocrine Review 2005; 16–21.

15 Nagelkerk J, Reick K, Meengs L. Perceived barriers and effective strategies to diabetes self-management. J Adv Nurs 2006; 54:151–158.

16 Glasgow RE, Hampson SE, Strycker LA, et al. Personal-model beliefs and social-environmental barriers related diabetes self-management. Diabetes Care 1997; 20:556–561.

17 Lauritzen T, Zoffmann V. Understanding the psychological barriers to effective diabetes therapy. Diabetes Voice 2004; 49:16–18.

18 Bayliss EA, Steiner JF, Fernald DH, et al. Descriptions of barriers to self-care by persons with comorbid chronic diseases. Ann Fam Med 2003; 1:15–21.

19 Ciechanowski PS, Katan WJ, Russo JE. Depression and diabetes. Arch Intern Med 2000; 160:3278–3285.

20 Polonsky WH, Earles J, Christensen R, et al. Integrating medical management with diabetes self-management training. Diabetes Care 2003; 26:3048–3053.

21 Nwasuruba C, Khan M, Egede LE. Racial/ethnic differences in multiple self-care behaviors in adults with diabetes. J Gen Intern Med 2007; 22:115–120.

22 Sarkar U, Fisher L, Schillinger D. Is self-efficacy associated with diabetes self-management across race/ethnicity and health literacy? Diabetes Care 2006; 29:823–829.

23 Aljasem LI, Peyrot M, Wissow L, et al. The impact of barriers and self-efficacy on self-care behaviors in type 2 diabetes. Diabetes Educ 2001; 27:393–404.

24 Polonsky WH. Encouraging effective self-management in diabetes. US Endocrine Disease 2006. Available at: www.touchbriefings.com/cdps/cditem.cfm?nid=1815&cid=5. Last accessed September 2007.

25 Del Prato S, Felton AM, Munro N, et al; Global Partnership for Effective Diabetes Management. Improving glucose management: ten steps to get more patients with type 2 diabetes to glycaemic goal. Int J Clin Pract 2005; 59:1345–1355.

26 Funnell M, Anderson RM. Empowerment and self-management of diabetes. Clinical Diabetes 2004; 22:123–127.

Index

Abbreviations

DPP-IV	dipeptidyl peptidase IV
DREAM	Diabetes REduction Assessment with ramipril and rosiglitazone Medication
GAD	glutamic acid decarboxylase
GLP-1	glucagon-like peptide 1
NPH	neutral protamine Hagedorn
STOP-NIDDM	Study To Prevent Non-Insulin-Dependent Diabetes Mellitus
TRIPOD	Troglitazone in the Prevention of Diabetes

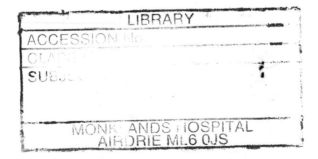